Tell Me the Planets

Tell Me the Planets

Stories of Brain Injury and
What It Means to Survive

BEN PLATTS-MILLS

FIG TREE
an imprint of
PENGUIN BOOKS

FIG TREE

UK | USA | Canada | Ireland | Australia
India | New Zealand | South Africa

Fig Tree is part of the Penguin Random House group of companies
whose addresses can be found at global.penguinrandomhouse.com.

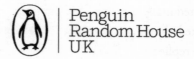

First published 2018
001

Permissions: photograph on page 107 of Harvey Cushing from the Wellcome Library and
contrast-enhanced magnetic resonance angiography of the carotid arteries on page 66 from Magnetic
Resonance Technology Information Portal, http://www.mr-tip.com

Illustration on page 22 by Rachael Tremlett

Set in 12/14.75 pt Bembo Book MT Std
Typeset by Jouve (UK), Milton Keynes
Printed in Great Britain by Clays Ltd, St Ives plc

A CIP catalogue record for this book is available from the British Library

ISBN: 978–0–241–25721–0

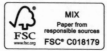

I paused and flipped through a *National Geographic* on the table. 'Tell me the planets,' I said, 'and something about them.' Unhesitatingly, confidently, he gave me the planets – their names, their discovery, their distance from the sun, their estimated mass, character, and gravity.

'What is this?' I asked, showing him a photo in the magazine I was holding.
'It's the moon,' he replied.
'No, it's not,' I answered. 'It's a picture of the earth taken from the moon.'
'Doc, you're kidding! Someone would've had to get a camera up there!'
'Naturally.'
'Hell! You're joking – how the hell would you do that?'

Oliver Sacks, 'The Lost Mariner' (1984)

I picture a classroom. Its dimensions are like one I remember from primary school but the light is different – reddish and somehow dark, as though the room sits inside a body. It is silent. There is the soft, bitter smell of pencil shavings. I know there would have been others here, but I can only see one person. He sits at his desk, motionless. His head is dark and perfectly round, his small shoulders dressed in a thin white shirt. Moving closer, I kneel at the side of his desk. A ghost here, I watch as he carefully transcribes the statements that have been written on the blackboard into his copybook. And I begin to feel his thoughts. This almost certainly never happened. It is a memory that should not exist. But I believe it to be true.

A person may fly like a bird.

The boy understands that this, like so much at school, is a kind of test. Like other tests, it has the structure of a trap. There is no way, perfectly, to know what is being asked. Humans may certainly fly. The boy knows that he has flown himself – that time, as a baby – though he does not remember it. But the word 'like' is troublesome, a hard little knot in the string of the sentence. 'Like a bird' may mean many things, only some of which are true when applied to human flight – by use of feathers, by flapping, in solitude, without mechanical assistance. But he also knows there is only one way forward: with courage. He writes: *Sometimes true.*

Snakes are poisonous.

It is 1987. The boy is nine years old. But what this means he can't entirely say. Time, for him, has not yet distinguished itself from change – from the coursing of heat through his body, from the fresh custom of waking each day, the happy sting of air on his face and arms. There is, in a sense, no such thing as the boy, as yet. He cannot, yet, himself, be reliably described. When he thinks about a snake, of what are the boy's thoughts composed? Nobody knows.

Every question has an answer.

The children around him are quietly working. He sees one boy looking out of the classroom window. There are no answers out there, only earth and sun. Yes, these questions are designed to ensnare but there is something about them he finds seductive. If he is silent, if he treads softly, he can move around each one and observe without disturbing it. There is a space in his mind for this. And he is not made uncomfortable by the quietness required.

The earth moves around the sun.

In each case, he is tempted by twin but opposing rewards: that of answering truthfully, keeping faith with the extent of his own mind, and that of answering correctly, in the manner expected by his teacher. *The earth moves around the sun.* The answer expected by the teacher here is 'always true'. This is one of those concrete beliefs that schooling rests upon. Like the love of God, the sum of one plus one. But he has read of other things in his father's books: the ageing of the solar system over millennia, the final collapse of the star at its centre, the engulfing and destruction of the inner planets and the falling away of those at the perimeter. He knows he is taking too long. He may not finish the test. This often happens.

A human may turn into a stone.

It has not occurred to the boy – how could it? – that there is anything wrong with his hearing. He is aware of an imbalance, certainly. He has looked at his ears in the mirror at home, inserted a finger, cupped his hands to his head in order to funnel the sound of his voice – first to one ear, then to the other. The left one seems not to function as the other one does but, he rationalizes, people are either left- or right-handed. It's only natural that they should be left- or right-eared as well. It will be years from now when he is told that most people's ears are the same.

The leaves must fall from a tree.

Standing next to the boy, forgetting what I know outside this dream, I see that his future is undecided. Anything might happen, nothing can be known. Nevertheless, there are things already in place – things that, though they cannot define him entirely, may pre-dispose him to certain kinds of action, or inaction; may with time prove persistent and be confirmed as the characteristics for which he is considered by others to be distinct, vivid, intractable. He is suspicious of his bodily urges, captivated by the patterns of his mind, relentlessly argumentative and pedantic to the point of banality. He is also sensitive, gentle, compassionate, conscientious and fiercely loyal. He has a highly developed sense of justice that can have come not from any teaching but rather only from his own determination of the facts. He is unusually abstract. There are some things that cannot be reduced: he will not be spoken to as a child; he willingly accepts solitude over any kind of compromised companionship. Even as a nine-year-old he is hard-minded.

It's a long way off, but with hindsight one can see those qualities that predisposed him to a career in computers – literacy and literality, a love of concision and accuracy, rigour. These may also be the qualities that equip him to pursue a path of self-determination, to build a life through the application of will. He will cope better than most with uncertainty. Though his emotions will challenge him as much as any person's might, his steadiness of mind, his commitment to reason, will help him to contain them when necessary, to wait things out and avoid panic. Do these same qualities predispose him to an unusual tolerance of loss? Is he better prepared than others to cope as his life is destroyed by the fates, when the time comes? Hard to say.

All mammals have fur.

Are these qualities that arise from the idiosyncrasies of the body, from the filaments that float in the chemical waters inside us? Surely, yes, always true. But none can say how. For some propositions, like God, are both true and indescribable.

Every person is born.

I watch as the boy writes: *Sometimes true.* For some of us are cut from the womb by the hands of others.

2014

Monday 4 August. Matthew has been confabulating. It's something that happens when he's worried or stressed. He remembers things that haven't occurred, or mixes up the details. He goes to medical appointments and brings back conflicting messages – telling me the surgeons want to operate, telling me he wants them to operate, and then telling me they don't plan to operate at all. It's not clear what's going on, and this is an important decision. It strikes me that really the surgeons are unlikely to allow Matthew to *choose* to have surgery. I imagine they might let him opt out, but they won't be cutting into his brain again unless they think it's absolutely necessary.

We'd agreed some months ago that I would come along to his appointments this year, but then he emails me to say he will be late tomorrow because he has a brain scan in the morning. So I text him to remind him about our deal.

Matthew has scans every six months or so, and the latest ones suggest that the cyst which was removed from his brain back in 2005 may be regrowing.

He texts me back:

> No problem. I'll meet you at
> the hospital at 8.15am.

The next day at the hospital reception he announces, 'I'm here to see a Mr Gadolinium.'

He's deadpan, but he's making a joke. He holds the letter out. 'It says, MRI appointment with Gadolinium.'

The man at the desk laughs. 'Gadolinium is the contrast agent.'

'Ah, *Agent* Gadolinium. So that's who I'm seeing.'

Down the corridor, we are in the future. This is the medical bay on the Starship *Enterprise*. The MRI scanner glows in soft yellow light beyond the window in the door. Matthew is inside, being injected with the agent.

A sleepy-eyed man in Crocs is changing the water jugs in the waiting room. His tag says his name is Victor. His job title is Imaging Assistant. I ask him what he knows about MRI. He says it takes about half an hour. I ask about the injection. He says yes, the contrast agent. 'Gadolinium is like turning on a light inside you,' he says. 'It makes it easier to see.'

When Victor is gone again I stand up. Through the window I can see the technician in charge of the machine. She has a greyscale image on a screen in front of her that shows a view of the top of Matthew's head from a camera mounted at the far end of the scanner. He's in there, being lit up from the inside.

Afterwards, we are walking back towards the tube station when Matthew spots a man with tattoos all up his arms. 'Oh, man, I wish I had tattoos like that.' He's never said this before. I'm surprised. 'But I couldn't do it. It would really freak my parents out. Maybe if I had a good job and a big salary and I could just say "whatever" to them.'

'What would you have a tattoo of?'

'Just an abstract pattern. Like the Maoris. They have some of the best tattoos.'

He's quiet for a moment, then, 'No, wait – I'd have an algorithm. Just a really simple algorithm like a factorial.'

'What's a factorial?'

'It's *n* times *n*-minus-one times *n*-minus-two – all the way down to one.'

'And again in English?'

He thinks for a moment.

'It's the number of ways you can choose from a set of things. So if for example you have three different-coloured balls. Take the first one. How many ways can you select that item?'

'One?'

'Exactly. And if you have two different-coloured balls, how many ways can you select *them*?'

I have no idea what he's talking about.

'You have two separate choices to start off with,' he says.

'Four?' I venture.

'Two . . . times . . . ?' He thinks I should know the answer.

'What do you mean, "how many ways can you select them?"' I say.

'How many different ways can you select them or arrange them?'

'Well, you could choose the . . . red one first?'

'Yes.'

'Or the green one first.'

'So you have two choices. Then after choosing that one, you have how many choices left?'

'Just don't choose any of them.'

'No, you have one choice left. So it's two times one.'

'So it's two.'

'Yeah. Two choices to select two things. And if you have *three* things, how many ways do you have? You have the first choice of three, times the choice of how you pick two things. Right?'

I'm lost.

'Because you know how to pick two things, right? So if you're going to pick three things – just say, "Well, I can either pick one, two, three." Then after that, you have to pick two things again. Which you already know. So it would be three times two factorial.' He looks at me, waiting for my agreement. 'Because you know how to pick two things, right?' he prompts.

'You know how to pick two things?'

'Yes. Already. That's two times one. So if you're going to pick three things . . .'

'Six?' (I am totally guessing.)

'Yeah. Then four factorial would be four options times three factorial. And that's how you calculate it. It's silly maths. But for functional programming it's really interesting. Ugh, I can taste it now.'

'The gadolinium?'

'It tastes like – urrgh . . .'

'What does it taste like?'

'Phlegm. It tastes like phlegm. But not on your tongue. At the back of your throat.'

'What language would you have your tattoo in?'
'Lisp or Haskell.'

Some Internet research later on reveals that, dating from 1958, Lisp is the second-oldest high-level programming language still in common use. Haskell is a lot more recent. It's what's known as a 'lazy functional language' – one that enables a lot of clever shortcuts, apparently. I text Matthew:

> Would it be fair to say Lisp is an old-school choice, while Haskell is more of a fast car – something a bit more techy?

He replies:

> Yup. Very right.

> Lisp is something rather special though. Imagine a spoken language wherein you could create new grammatical forms as you speak. Awesome, no?

I've known Matthew for eight years – almost as long as I've been working at Headway, the charity where he and I met in 2006, the year after his brain injury. Until then Matthew had been a software engineer. He can still program in C++ and Java. He holds a degree in Maths and Computer Science from University College London. He is one of the brainiest people I know.

It's like turning on a light inside you, Victor the Imaging Assistant had said. The gadolinium, illuminating you from the inside. It makes me think of the crest on the gates of St Leonard's Church in Shoreditch, a hundred yards from where Headway used to be. It's in the shape of a shield. On a red background there is a pair of seated gold lions with their front paws raised and touching. Their faces meet and join somehow in the middle – the right side attached to one body, the left to the other. Below the Siamese twins is a curly scroll on which are written the words *More Light, More Power.*

It dates from the turn of the last century, when the neighbourhood was a notorious slum and the local authority became the first in London to introduce electric street lighting. The lights would reduce crime, it was thought. Not far away, on Old Street, Shoreditch Town Hall features a facade from the same period, including a statue carrying an axe and a flaming torch, beneath which, in large letters, the word *PROGRESS* is cut into the stone. Clear the way, shine the light.

This memory feels autumnal: it must be 2006 or 2007, around the time Matthew first came to Headway. I'm out for a walk with one of the clients: Sid. Sid and I get on. I admire him. He seems to have a sense of humour, despite everything. In some ways, of course, it's a one-sided friendship. I don't know what, if anything, he thinks of me.

Of the people you could meet at Headway, he definitely isn't the one that would strike you as looking the worst off. He is pale and unkempt. His clothes are inexpensive – tracksuit bottoms, ill-fitting shirts. He walks oddly, like an old man, shuffling along. If you get closer, you notice a long vertical fault line beneath the skin of his forehead, running up from his left eye into his thinning hair. But others are more noticeably scarred, like Mike, whose injury and subsequent surgery left him with a huge indentation that takes up almost half his head and which he covers most of the time with a hat. And Sid has a degree of physical function that others lack: he has the use of both arms, his hands are warm and his grip is strong. He can do things – like the washing-up – and can take himself to the toilet. He's good at chess and rummy.

But Sid's outward completeness disguises a profound loss. There is a space inside him where things go in and never come out again.

We've gone for the walk because he was getting annoyed. He wants to smoke all the time but he can't do it indoors and he'd just be

at the front entrance all day if we didn't try to distract him – and he
enjoys other things once he gets into them, like walking. We're making our way down the concrete ramp at the front, into the courtyard.
I'm asking him what he used to do for work. I've asked him before,
probably fifteen times, but I'm asking him again to see if he says anything different. He seems to like reminiscing. He has a nice way of
going about a conversation, as far as it goes. He's gentle, matter of fact.

'I worked in a bank.'

'Which one?'

'Barclays.'

'Did you like it?'

'Not much. I left after a couple of years.' Sid speaks quietly, with a
husky voice from all the smoking. He mumbles a bit. To my ear he
also sounds slightly northern, Lancastrian perhaps. He flattens his
vowels. As I understand it, he has always lived in London, apart from
trips abroad.

'What did you do next?'

'I went to Israel.' This is all the same as before. I know he worked
on a kibbutz. He met French girls there. He didn't work that hard. I
ask him all the same.

'What did you do there?'

'I worked on a kibbutz.'

'How long for?'

'About a year.'

'Did you work hard?'

'Not really, after I'd been there a while.'

Once we get to the bottom of the slope, I ask which way he wants
to go. He looks each way and gestures ahead of us. We walk into the
courtyard. There are big loading-bay doors at the end that belong to
the Mildmay Hospital. Sometimes lorries reverse in here, beeping.
There's a skip with bits of wood in it, a white door off its hinges.
Next to that there's an old washing machine waiting for collection,
some black metal dustbins as tall as me.

'What can you see, Sid?' I ask.

Sid pauses and looks ahead. After a moment he says, 'Farming
equipment.'

We make our way over to the other side of the courtyard.

'What can you see now?'

'Tractor.'

He's looking at a big London plane tree in front of us, its flaky bark like a jigsaw. Sid's memories of Israel are bleeding into the present day, I think. His vision is a jumble – he is seeing what he is thinking about. Can that be so?

'Why don't you touch it, Sid?'

He puts out his hand, leaning forward a bit, his feet staying rooted to the spot. He looks like a person in the dark, searching for the light switch. His fingertips touch the bark. He strokes the rough surface a little. 'A tree.'

We walk gradually out of the front gates and up Austin Street towards the churchyard. Sid asks if he can have a cigarette.

'I haven't got any on me, Sid. They're back at the centre.'

'Can we go back now?'

'Yeah, if you like. Or we could just have a look at the churchyard and then go back.'

'OK.'

As we approach, I can see a man sitting on one of the benches over by the church. He has a can in his hand. There are more big plane trees here, hissing in the breeze. The church is dilapidated, the sunlight showing the dirt on the windowpanes behind the wire grilles.

We enter by the north-east gate, past the lions on the shield, and stop by the flowerbeds.

'What can you see now, Sid?'

His face is very white, almost the colour of wax. Little black hairs poke out of it. His eyes are very black too, like river stones.

'Farming instruments. A tractor.'

A scatter of pigeons fly overhead towards Calvert Avenue, their wings clattering. It smells like earth and rust here. The man on the bench shifts, takes a drink from his can. He looks over at us.

I look at the flowers. Sid looks at them too.

'What colours can you see, Sid?'

His eyes flicker. 'Dark red,' he says. 'White?'

I point at the yellow flowers. 'What colours here?'

'Orange? Red?'

Sid looks at me. 'Can I have a cigarette?'

'They're back at the centre.'

'Can we go back now?'

'Of course.'

I watch as Sid turns and shuffles back the way we came. At first he's going the right way, but when he gets to the gate he goes to turn left, down Austin Street, away from Headway. He doesn't seem too tired or anxious. Maybe he has changed his mind about the cigarette. I catch up with him and we walk together along the church railings, in the direction of Hackney Road. The man on the bench inside the churchyard watches us. A blackbird lands on the railings just ahead. It watches us too, its black eye inside a perfect yellow ring.

Sid pauses. 'Where are we going, sir?' He often calls me sir.

'I'm not sure, Sid. Where do you think we are?'

'Israel?'

'No.'

'France?'

France is where Sid went after his time in Israel. He's told me about it before. Picking grapes.

'No, we're in London,' I say. 'France was a long time ago, Sid. Nearly thirty years.'

'That is a long time ago.'

Sid never seems too upset by his disorientation. I get the sense that it rarely occurs to him to wonder where he is, or notice that he has no idea. If I ask him the question when we are at the centre he usually says Whipps Cross Nuthouse or Whipps Cross Prison. I suppose Whipps Cross must have been local to him at some stage. I suppose there must be some vague sense on his part that his liberty is being impinged on – that he's not quite free these days. Hence the institutional guesses. Or maybe it's the company. It's mostly men at Headway. A couple of the more vocal ones have been in prison.

Sometimes if he's anxious Sid will say he needs to go home. When you ask him why, he says to feed Auntie, his cat. At first I assumed he might have been right – maybe he did have a cat at home. But Auntie is dead – she's been dead a long time, apparently. Sid lives in a nursing home now, no pets allowed. He's thinking about a time before his injury, when he lived with his brother. If you ask him about it, he'll tell you. His brother, the cat, his mum. If you ask Sid how old he is he'll say thirty-six. He's forty-four.

He got his injury eight years ago. His notes say he was found unconscious in the car park outside a pub, bleeding from his head. His skull was fractured and there was a lot of blood inside. His brain had been crushed by the initial blow and by the build-up of blood that could not escape. Nobody knows what happened. It might have been a mugging. Later, when he was unconscious in hospital, he began fitting very badly. The doctors were worried that the seizures would cause further brain damage. They had established that the fits were coming from the most damaged part of his brain, the left frontal lobe. They took off the front part of his skull and removed the lobe – about a fifth of his brain.

'Who am I, Sid?'

'You're Paul.'

'Who's Paul?'

'My best friend in the world.'

'How did you meet him?'

'We worked together. Can I have a cigarette?'

'Yes. They're back at the centre though, that way.' I point behind him. He turns around. We begin the walk back. We pass a blue door. A white one. We turn into the courtyard and Sid pauses again. He asks for a cigarette. I tell him we're on our way to get one.

'Sid.'

'Yes?'

'What's our relationship? You and me?'

'You're my boss.'

'I'm not your boss.'

'Fellow worker?'

'No.'

We are at the front door. The sun shines on the concrete slope. A trail of smoke moves along the bricks above the ashtray on the wall ahead of us.

'We're at Headway,' I say. 'It's a place that looks after people who've had accidents.'

Sid looks at me.

'Have I had an accident?'

I'm not sure how to answer this. I hadn't expected it. Will he get upset if I say yes? Will he be able to understand? He doesn't say anything, just looks at me, waiting for an answer. After another moment he smiles.

'What does that mean?' he asks, tapping his knuckles on the side of his head as if to show there's nothing in there. Then he laughs and puts out a hand for me to shake. He has a strong grip. His hand is dry. He's enjoying the joke. It's no big deal.

He looks at me and takes a slow breath.

'Can I have a cigarette?'

★

Friday 10 October. I'm expecting to see Matthew waiting for me at the tube station. I can recognize him a mile off. He almost always wears the same jacket – a blue-and-black cycling waterproof. His skin is dark. He has a round head and large, soft hands; an unassuming posture. And he has a habit of being early. When he puts appointments in his phone he usually subtracts at least half an hour from the actual meeting time, in case of delays. But as I step off my bike there's no sign of him. I take my phone from my pocket and call him.

'Hello?'

'Hey Matthew, where are you?'

'I'm at the, ah . . .' There's a pause. I imagine him looking around for the name. 'I'm in reception.' He's already there.

'OK, I'll see you in two minutes.'

He's standing in the lobby, facing the doors, drinking from a little white cup as I walk in. He waves and smiles. He looks tired. This is another unchanging quality – he always looks tired.

We're told to go up to the second floor and wait to be called.

This is a private hospital. Its website describes its on-site pathology lab, its laminar-flow operating theatres, whatever they are, its recently upgraded £1.6 million cardiac catheterization suite. It's somewhere you go if you've got money and don't want to muck about with the NHS (Matthew doesn't have money – we're here as visitors rather than patients). It also has some of the most advanced CT scanners in the country.

Matthew rummages in his bag. 'One of my trusty thirty-two-gig memory sticks,' he says as he pulls out a small rectangle of plastic and hands it to me. I'm going to record the meeting we are here for; Matthew has brought the USB stick so that I can save the audio file on to it for him.

'You know,' says Matthew, 'there was a time when if you had a thirty-two-gig memory in your computer you were doing really well.' He laughs, acknowledging the absurdity of the idea. How things change.

I turn the memory stick over in my hand and wonder how much memory a CT scanner has. I drop it into the small pocket on the front of my backpack and do up the zip.

And then Mr Hau appears in front of us. The man we are here to meet. The man who gave Matthew brain damage.

'If I remember correctly, it was the headache, wasn't it?' Mr Hau is trying to recall Matthew's condition when he first saw him back in 2005. He says he's seen hundreds of patients in the intervening years. 'Or was it the double vision?'

The symptoms sound innocent enough, but in Matthew's case they were signs of acute obstructive hydrocephalus, a potentially fatal condition caused when something prevents the drainage of fluid from the brain's ventricles. By the time Mr Hau saw him, I understand, Matthew was in a critical condition. The surgery to remove the blockage – a growth known as a colloid cyst – saved his life.

Mr Hau speaks softly. He's warm and funny and takes an immediate interest in Matthew's progress. As we settle at the desk in his small consulting room he asks how Matthew is physically. Is everything OK work-wise? How are his mental powers? He listens carefully to the answers and quickly begins to seek more detail when Matthew confesses he remains out of work and significantly cognitively impaired.

'How bad is the memory?' asks Mr Hau. 'Say 100 per cent is normal. How many per cent are you?'

'Oh,' Matthew considers. 'Mine is less than . . .' he looks at me, 'thirty?'

I know plenty of people with worse memories than Matthew, but they generally don't live independently. In terms of independence, Matthew is right on the cusp. He gets by, but life is a struggle.

Mr Hau says the amnesia is a consequence of the surgery – it became evident shortly after Matthew came round from the operation.

This is what we're here for: clarity. It's now nine years since the operation, and for much of that time Matthew has been floundering – hoping his impairments will improve, trying to work out if the cyst is still causing problems, researching whether he might need repeat surgery. Mr Hau isn't Matthew's doctor any more, but he's been kind enough to make time for us all the same.

He tells us how the surgery to remove a colloid cyst works.

'We make a small window in the surface of the brain,' he says. 'We stretch the opening and go down and then we reach the water cavity in the middle of the brain. From there we can see the cyst very well and take it out.

'But,' he continues, 'during your surgery, when we took out the cyst, maybe we stretched the memory fibres.'

Can he be more specific? What brain structures is he referring to?

'The fornices,' he says, 'or maybe the mammillary bodies.'

He tells us that success rates for colloid cyst surgery are generally good. The majority of patients do not experience cognitive impairment afterwards.

Matthew explains that for him the memory impairment is less important than the fatigue. The fatigue is what stops him living a normal life. Mr Hau asks him to elaborate – physical fatigue, mental? Matthew says he's not sure. 'I mean, I feel it physically. Sometimes my bones just ache. If I can overcome the fatigue,' he says, 'then I think I would be perfectly fine in holding down a job, as long as I used my memory techniques.'

Then Matthew tells Mr Hau about his most recent brain scan: it showed that the cyst had regrown by a few millimetres. 'Oh, no,' says Mr Hau.

Matthew says he has had some conflicting advice: when he saw the registrar after the scan, he was told he should have repeat surgery. But then, later, when he saw his consultant, he was told this was not a good option.

Mr Hau tries to clarify. 'It's maybe not big enough yet. You can always ask to see your consultant and he can explain.'

'I wrote to him,' says Matthew, 'but I didn't get a reply.'

'Oh, they are very busy,' says Mr Hau, 'it's difficult. But anyway, surgery has risks. They don't operate unless the cyst is causing a problem. Colloid cysts tend to be asymptomatic. In many people they are only found accidentally or as an emergency – when it's become very serious. Fatigue isn't usually a symptom.'

He pauses for a moment, thinking, and then tells us that the father of neurosurgery, Harvey Cushing, had a colloid cyst. 'He worked twenty-four hours a day. No fatigue! His cyst was only found in the post-mortem.'

Mr Hau tries to help us understand how fraught neurosurgical decision-making can be, how hard it is to assess the likely impact on each patient.

'Someone who is normal cognitively,' he says, 'starting with a cognitive power of 100 per cent – if you drop that by 5, 10 per cent, the guy would still be independent, yes? Able to work, et cetera. He's still functioning. Someone who is teetering on the edge, say 50 per cent, then you drop it down to less than 50, suddenly he becomes jobless. So although the risk is very similar, in terms of the person the consequence is very, very different. If you have 100 per cent you can afford to lose a little bit. But if you are poor then you can't even afford to lose the pennies.'

I have never come across this economic metaphor before, this quantity theory of cognition, but it makes a lot of sense. You can understand how a brain surgeon would be looking for ways to make the discussion of risk as concrete as possible.

Before his surgery, Matthew was a Harvey Cushing. A 100-per-center. A sixty-hour-week high-achiever. Maybe if he'd been referred when his cyst had been smaller, discovered by accident because of a scan for something else, this is how the discussion would have gone: in terms of percentages, costs and benefits. I can see Matthew dealing with this well, given his love of numbers, his disciplined thinking.

'Paradoxically,' says Mr Hau, 'emergencies are much easier because if we don't do anything you die. There's not so much debating.'

But survival isn't the only consideration. 'There's the query about the state of the patient in the long term, whether you're going to be independent, self-caring. That's the difficult bit.'

And how is that assessed?

'You just have to do your best based on your feeling and on what the team feels, what the family feels. You can't know what will be a life worth living for the patient.'

To illustrate this point, Mr Hau talks about a paper he read some years ago: a study in which people with spina bifida were asked to imagine that a cure for their disabilities had been discovered. Spina bifida is a long-term spinal condition that comes with a raft of complex problems: mobility and learning impairments, problems with continence, scoliosis and back pain. In the scenario given to the study participants, Mr Hau explains, the imaginary cure would completely remove all of their symptoms with the only side effect being that they would lose a week of their life expectancy.

'Guess how many people said yes,' says Mr Hau. 'Only about 40 per cent! And then they asked them, if they knew they were going to pass on the condition to their children would they still have children? How many said yes? Eighty per cent. One characteristic of humans is their ability to adapt. If you're standing on the outside you say, "Oh my God, compared to my life, this is terrible," but, you know, people don't want *your* life. You have to ask people. You have to ask your patients what's important to them.'

He turns to Matthew. 'What's most important? For me my memory's most important, but you say fatigue is more important than memory. What a surprise. For memory you can use methods to compensate. In all walks of life there are people with good memories, people with bad memories, but they're still living their lives. Fatigue's more difficult to compensate for. You don't have tricks to make you not feel tired. Red Bull maybe!'

'One of the tricks I've learned,' says Matthew, 'that doesn't actually work.'

'The problem with brain injury,' says Mr Hau, 'is that you damage the organ that helps you to adapt to your new situation.'

I look at Matthew. He says only, 'Yes.'

★

The place where Mr Hau cut through Matthew's scalp is plainly visible: a pair of half-moon scars just below the hairline, either side of the widow's peak. They catch the light like trails of water when Matthew looks down at his phone, or at his feet.

The cyst is a pearl of fatty tissue that grows from the roof of the third ventricle in the centre of the brain. About one person in every 20,000 has one, but most are asymptomatic, causing no more harm than a mole or a crooked tooth. Many people, like Harvey Cushing, live and die never knowing the cyst was there. The dangerous ones are the ones that grow.

The ventricles produce about a pint of cerebral spinal fluid per day, suspending the brain in a constantly renewed bath of salty water. A large cyst can obstruct the openings through which the fluid drains,

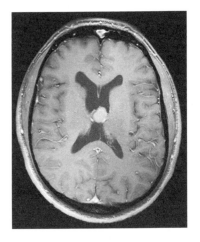
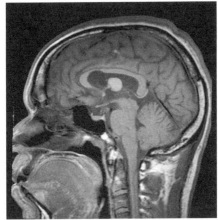

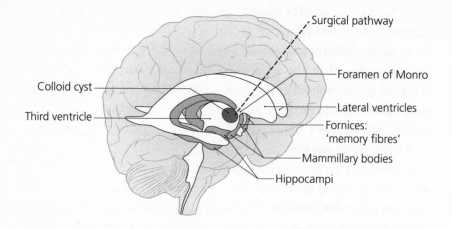

turning the ventricles into fluid-filled balloons that threaten to crush the brain against the inside of the skull. As pressure builds, the optic nerves begin to get squashed, causing the blurred vision Matthew experienced as his earliest symptom. Headaches set in as the nerves and blood vessels around the brain are constricted and, as things get worse, blackouts start to occur. If the blockage isn't removed quickly, sudden death is a distinct possibility.

From the diagrams I find on the Internet it appears that both the fornices and the mammillary bodies, the structures described by Mr Hau as the 'memory fibres', are embedded in the limbic system – a strange and ancient neural territory at the centre of the brain that has significant roles in memory and emotion. It looks as though the fornices in particular are intimately connected to the hippocampi, forming another branch of their horn-like structure.

I think of Henry Molaison, one of the most famous amnesiacs in the psychology literature, who had most of both of his hippocampi removed in a misguided attempt to cure his epilepsy, with devastating effects on his ability to form new memories. From his late twenties onwards he lived much of his life in a scientific institute under close watch, earning his keep as a research subject.

The mammillary bodies appear to sit somewhere towards the foremost ends of the fornices.

It's hard to get an idea of how the separate structures relate to one another, but I slowly arrive at the understanding that the voids between the different parts of the limbic system – the negative spaces – are none other than the fluid-filled ventricles. The third ventricle, inside which the colloid cyst grows, is separated from the lateral ventricles above by the fornices. Its floor is made out of the mammillary bodies. The memory fibres are the very walls of this cave, the very stuff from which the cyst has grown.

During the interview we had asked Mr Hau what kinds of conditions were most amenable to brain surgery. He had given his gentle laugh and said, 'Ones that don't involve the brain.' Problems occurring in the spaces around the brain were generally quite easy to address, he had said: malformations in the blood supply, cancers of the surrounding membranes. 'But anything to do with the brain tissue itself, like tumour of the brain, then we do very badly. Hopefully in the next fifty years we will eventually get better. But so far we are very good at everything but the brain.'

The cyst is not brain tissue, but to get to it you must go through the brain. Collateral damage, then.

Technology brings us magic. It brings us the illusion of plenty, of permanence. It brings us life after death.

For most of human history, people with significant brain injuries tended to die, but with the introduction of scanning technology like Magnetic Resonance Imaging (MRI) and Computed Tomography (CT) in the 1970s the game changed. Suddenly illuminated, the inside of the skull was now accessible to targeted treatment, and survival rates began to surge.

But as powerful as our technologies become there remains one problem they cannot solve: that of human frailty. However well guided, brain surgery for illnesses like Matthew's carries with it the high risk of permanent damage. And a good proportion of trauma patients – those injured, like Sid, in accidents and fights – have non-fatal but disabling brain injuries. So, in working its magic, medicine has given rise to a new population. Those who would previously have died now live, in many cases, a natural term, with complex neurological impairments. In the absence of adequate support as many as 80 per cent of these survivors experience mental health problems, many are isolated and 70 per cent are long-term unemployed. The suicide rate for survivors is four times that of the general population.

*

Matthew and I leave Mr Hau's office and walk down the main street until we find a cafe. We sit at a table on the wide pavement and order coffee. I spent years telling Matthew to drink less coffee, on the basis that reduced caffeine intake would improve his sleep, but I've given up now. It doesn't seem to matter what Matthew does: the fatigue remains a stubborn mystery.

There's a poster for a film about the Bullingdon Club on the wall nearby. Matthew says he wants to see it. It's useful to know about these things, he says. These people run the country. We talk about politics, about TV, about Marxism. Then, after a pause, Matthew switches to something more personal:

'That volunteer,' he says, 'what's his name, Luke? He's really hot.'

Luke is German, gay and, yes, hot. He's been volunteering with Headway for a few months and has made a lot of friends. But this doesn't explain Matthew's behaviour – he has been going on about Luke like this for some weeks now.

'You know that quite a few people think you might be gay now, don't you?' I say. 'Sarah asked me if you were gay.'

'Yes, but he's really hot. He's so buff.'

Matthew laughs. I know he isn't gay. We have had numerous conversations about the women he has, in one way or another, been involved with; about his dilemmas over love – unrequited, abortive, impossible.

'Are you going to let me in on the secret?' I ask him.

'Well, when I first met Luke I realized I had some homophobic feelings. So I thought about it and I asked myself what would be the best way to put myself in his shoes. So I understood the best way was to make some people think I might be gay. That way I would know better what it was like to actually be gay, to be Luke, and I would hopefully be able to get rid of those prejudices.'

I'm lost for words. It's this kind of thing, more than anything, that makes me admire Matthew. He is, despite everything, and more so than anyone I know, committed to clarity, to honesty, to a life of reason. He is determined to confront the world – and himself within it – as it is given. He is determined to root out and relinquish his ungenerous instincts. However demanding his own circumstances might be, however exhausting, he is determined to be a human striving for greater humanity.

Matthew has told me before: what has made life bearable since his injury is other people. Before, he was a loner, an introvert, a person of rugged self-sufficiency. But since that day he woke in hospital, that self-sufficiency has been tested to its limits. He has learned that independence is merely a euphemism for having good friends or no enemies. He sees the role of luck in life. And he sees every day the evidence of the hard work behind the modern fantasy of effortless consumerism: the bus drivers, the street sweepers, the greengrocers; and he thinks about the invisible people – the data-enterers, the helpline technicians, the thousands standing under far-off strip lights packing parcels at the Amazon warehouses.

If he could, he would go back to work, I know. He's tried many times over the years.

I think again about the spina bifida study Mr Hau had referred to. I ask Matthew how many years he would be willing to sacrifice for a cure to his cognitive impairments.

'I'd trade five years,' he says. 'A decade is too much.'

He thinks a moment. 'But it's not that simple because there are many experiences you could have in those five years that may not be worth a cure. And it depends what you'd do with the rest of your life with your healthy mind.'

'And what would you do with your healthy mind?'

'I'd be working six days a week,' he says, and starts laughing.

The life that medical technology has given Matthew is not the life he chose – the one in which he was in control, in which he was master of his own destiny. The life technology has given Matthew is full of anxiety, full of fear. He is, every day, acutely aware of his own mortality. Matthew, more than most, sees the world for what it is: a precious thing for which we are each responsible, a thing we each stand to lose at a moment's notice through neglect or carelessness or a stroke of bad luck.

★

Even now, after more than a decade, every day when I arrive at work I have a good feeling. I don't enjoy everything about my job. I spend too much time at a desk, and sadly these days I'm based across the road from the main centre, a little isolated from the action. But I always check in first thing, if only to sign the register and get a feel of the place while it's still quiet.

The members and volunteers start to arrive at about half past nine, and by eleven the place is heaving. Most days of the week we're at capacity, with up to fifty people in attendance, all told. The centre occupies the ground floor of a residential block on the Regent's Canal in Hackney, just where it intersects with Kingsland Road. It has a kitchen, a gym, some therapy rooms, offices, and a main space with tables where people spend a lot of their time talking and playing games. It also has a canal-side garden and an art studio in an adjacent railway arch, underneath the East London Line. We're too big for the place really. But nobody complains when there aren't enough seats at lunchtime.

We work with some of the most disabled, most disadvantaged people in the city and, with a catchment that covers some of the poorest boroughs in the UK, many of the most hard-up too. Because there are no other comparable services, we cover more than a third of the capital – everything above the river from Westminster as far north as Enfield and as far east as Dagenham. People travel for up to two hours to get to the centre. Many have told me it's the only place they can relax. For a few short hours in the week, they feel like they don't have to explain themselves or pretend to be anything they're not.

On a typical day you'll find Esi in the kitchen, making scones or bread and butter pudding with Pete, the baker. You'll find Henry in the studio, drawing a picture of a girl with three breasts, or a fox with mad eyes wearing a suit (you can ask him why; he'll just say, 'Why not?'). Francis will be in his usual spot on the table just outside the kitchen, reading the paper, keeping an eye on everybody (he sees everything; sometimes it's like he can see through walls). Sadie will be playing pool with someone, her voice audible across the whole centre when she pots a ball: 'Yessssss! Ha ha ha!' And when she doesn't: 'I can't believe it!' Chao Xing will be helping Esi in the kitchen, or standing quizzically in the middle of the room after finishing a gym session, lost-seeming but not unhappy, as though listening to the room around her, until someone asks her what her plan is. Keith will be making endless cups of tea for anyone who asks, forgetting how many he's made that day, ever willing. The dominoes guys will be playing dominoes, the sofa guys will be on the sofa, the smokers will be smoking, and the newspaper guys will be on the table near the kitchen with Francis, talking about the football, or about some scandal in the news. These are the patterns of the day, the rhythms that grow out of people's habits and friendships – the things they bring and share.

That's why I have the good feeling: because Headway East London is a real place, a place with a culture, a place with soul – a place where everyone's pulling in the same direction. This is what we have built together. This is what protects us and what we have to protect.

★

I accompany Matthew to a follow-up meeting about the most recent MRI scans. The consultant looks at the images in the same vague way he had six months earlier and says the cyst has not grown and should be treated 'conservatively'. This means leave it alone.

Over the following months I watch Matthew going about his voluntary work at Headway – washing up in the kitchen, talking to members in the art studio – and I have the sense that something is changing in him. He seems more relaxed, as though maybe he is finally starting to accept what's happened.

In many respects Matthew's needs are as great as any of the funded clients, but as far as the social services are concerned he's not disabled enough to warrant our support. So much of what I offer to do with him is informal – the kind of thing you might do for a colleague or a friend who is in trouble. In return he has helped me develop some of Headway's most interesting work. In 2010 we received a grant to make a documentary film about life with brain injury. Together we recruited two other survivors to help us.

In terms of the demands placed on abstract thinking, filming and editing, it turns out, are probably second only to software engineering. You couldn't really pick a harder thing to try and do if you have memory or concentration impairments. We made a handful of films – one of them we even got paid for. But the toll it took on all of us was ridiculous. There were terrible arguments. There were tears. I tried to film some of our work process as it collapsed. The project ate itself.

I remember the day Matthew told me I had failed the group by giving up too easily. It took him a while to forgive me, I think. But it brought us closer together.

I begin interviewing another volunteer, Danny, for a new project. The plan is to publish life stories on the Internet as a way of raising awareness. A colleague interviews Matthew for the same project and together we draft the written accounts, handing them back to Danny and Matthew for corrections and new thoughts. Matthew and Danny are some of our longest-standing volunteers. They seem like a good place to start.

★

Back in early September. Matthew is waiting for me when I get to Euston station just before 11 a.m. We are on our way to Portmeirion, a little town on the north-west coast of Wales. We've been invited to speak at a music festival there. I'm excited about it but also a little nervous – Matthew has never been to a music festival before, never been camping before. Am I dragging him into something he'll resent or be confused by or find ridiculous? He has said he wants to do this and his sister approved of it when we last spoke. But on some level I'm taking a bit of a chance. Where we are going is a long way from home.

Over his shoulder are three bags: the black courier's bag he always carries plus a pair of large white plastic ones with drawstrings that say *Ride 100* on them – freebies from a sponsored cycle ride he did a couple of weeks ago.

'Is that all you're bringing?' I ask.

'It's just two days, right?'

'Yes, but that doesn't look like much.'

'I'm African, we're used to sleeping rough.'

'You don't have a travel bag?' I ask.

'No. No luggage.'

'What did you do when you went to see your parents?' This was last year – the first time Matthew had gone back to Nigeria in ten years.

'My sister lent me a bag.'

'You've got a toothbrush? A towel?'

'Yes. Are there going to be showers?'

'I would think so.'

We walk over to look at the departures board. The station is busy, even at this hour. Among the throng I can already spot a few festival-looking types with rucksacks and wellies, straw hats. We have twenty minutes before the train is due to leave, so we walk outside and sit down at one of the black benches that break up the dirty courtyard in front of the station. People are smoking in the sun.

A young woman approaches us, pushing a pair of large bins on a cart. She is dressed in blue overalls and an orange high-vis vest, all of it much too big for her slight frame. She can't be more than twenty. Her skin is a reddish gold, her hair black. Matthew says hello, asks her how it's going. She doesn't reply, just picks up the discarded newspaper that's lying on the table between us.

'Where do you think she's from?' I ask Matthew when she's gone. 'She looks South East Asian.'

'Malaysia, maybe?'

'Laos?'

We are guessing. We talk about migration. We talk about capitalism. We always talk about capitalism. It's one long conversation we've been having on and off for years. Today Matthew's line is that capitalism is the only kind of civilization that has worked, that can work in the long run, because it's flexible, it can adjust to new developments, it isn't held back by religion or other beliefs. He is saying he watched something recently about how Islam is a failed civilization because it combines religion and politics – a problem that has always caused civilizations to fail. I wonder if he has tried this on any Muslims. I wouldn't be surprised: he's not shy of an argument.

'I have to send you this link,' he says, as we walk along the platform and board the train. 'Did I send you the link about this guy yet? The Marxist?'

'I don't think so.'

'Man, Marx was a clever guy.'

'So I hear.'

'*Das Kapital* was basically a condensation of a hyper-abstraction of how an economy works. It's an abstraction of an abstraction.'

'Have you read it?'

'No, but I'm learning about it on YouTube. YouTube is a wonderful thing.' Since his injury, Matthew finds it hard to retain information. Books are difficult; Internet TV is easier.

We sit down at a table opposite one another. Next to me a young woman fiddles with her phone. Matthew asks after a few people at Headway, Sid in particular. They used to spend a lot of time together when Sid was at the centre. 'Is he well?'

I tell him I haven't seen him in a while.

'Did I send you that link to the Marxist guy?' Matthew asks after a pause. I'm used to his forgetting, his repeating. It happens at a steady rate most days.

'No.'

'Have to send you that. This guy is very clever.'

'OK, yes, send it.'

Matthew looks out of the window as the train pulls away from the station. The girl wants to charge her phone, but the electrical socket isn't working.

'I watch a lot of far-right videos on YouTube,' Matthew says.

'Why?'

The girl is ignoring us, or pretending to.

'The truth is important,' says Matthew.

'You mean you want to know what people are thinking?'

'The fact is that Western cultures are more successful. Anglo-Saxon people have done better. And brain size varies between races.'

'You're not serious?' I'm sure we've had this conversation before. This is one of Matthew's topics, one of his ways of baiting me and other liberal lefties. But he's also serious about it. He likes having a knotty question to chew over, likes a challenge.

'There's no point ignoring the facts,' he says.

'OK.' I look out of the window. Am I going to have this discussion with him? It makes me want to laugh – how good he is at pressing buttons.

He smiles and stares at me. 'Don't you think?'

'I think there's a number of questions I'd ask,' I say, 'like what you mean by "success".'

'Well, it's obvious, isn't it? I mean, *ka-ching*.' He rubs his thumb and fingers together.

'OK, fine. But then I'd want to know whether you accept the terms on which that success has been achieved. Take America. That's a successful country in financial terms, right?'

'Yes.'

'So in that instance I'd want to know whether or not you consider genocide and slavery acceptable terms on which to attain success?'

'OK' – he looks at the table – 'good point.'

'In all but a very few cases – maybe in all cases – successful cultures are the ones most willing to enslave and wipe out the populations of other cultures.' Matthew doesn't know it but this isn't my own argument. I'm borrowing from a friend in America.

'But the results speak for themselves. You can't argue with the results,' he says.

'But what are those results? Do you think people are happier? Inequality is almost as bad now as it has ever been. Do you consider that a mark of success?'

'I don't know. We have managed to extend our lives by many years.'

'That's true.'

The girl next to me says, 'Excuse me.' She wants to move seats. Maybe our conversation is driving her away.

'You know the richest people who ever lived were all medievals?' I say. 'They were all alive in the twelfth and thirteenth centuries.'

'Ah, really?'

'Yeah. It was a time in history when wealth was concentrated in incredibly few hands and everybody else was impoverished.'

'That makes sense. Some people are saying that's how it's becoming again. We are going back to a kind of global feudalism.'

'Yes. It's the same. Except now the serfs live in Third World countries.'

Outside the train there are softly undulating fields and dark green copses. A tractor moves up a slope, opening the chocolate-brown earth. I think it's Oxfordshire.

Matthew is looking too. 'I always wondered why British people go on holidays,' he says.

'Why?'

'Well, you have this. It's really beautiful. Why go to Spain?'

'It is lovely.'

The sky is hazy. The fields give way to woods. A wide, silver river swings across our view and disappears. I think about swimming, feeling the water against my chest. I'm going to swim at the festival if I can. Portmeirion is on the estuary of the River Dwyryd. I've seen pictures: great sand flats and steady tidal waters, wide as a lake.

'Ah,' says Matthew, 'you know apparently Einstein's brain was smaller than average.'

'So what does that say about your far-right facts?'

'He was an Ashkenazi Jew. Sigmund Freud was Ashkenazi. Franz Kafka. If you look at history, many of the most intelligent people have been Ashkenazi. There has to be something in it.'

'So now you're making the same point with different evidence?'

'It's worth a try.'

'Again your premises are questionable.'

'Please elaborate.'

★

Six hours later we arrive at the festival site, secluded in woodland, a short walk from the shore of the Dwyryd estuary.

A man called Joe shows us the performance area where we will give our talk tomorrow, the Hendrick's tent, then walks us to the staff camping area – a small field into which a great many tents have been crammed. Matthew and I have our pick because we're the first to arrive. I choose a small orange one; Matthew takes a slightly larger blue one not far away.

'I'm not going to be able to remember which one it is,' says Matthew. He's right. It's an anonymous tent in a field full of anonymous tents. An amnesiac's nightmare. We agree that we'll stick together tonight and make sure he gets back to the right one.

'Is there a Lottery shop nearby?' Matthew asks.

Joe looks dubious. 'I don't think so.'

'You don't play the Lottery, do you?' I ask Matthew.

'It's my only route out of poverty!'

'You're more likely to get hit by a meteorite than win the Lottery. You're more likely to get a brain injury!'

Matthew laughs and shrugs. 'But the adverts keep saying it could be me.'

On the way back to the main festival site, Joe asks Matthew about his injury.

'It was a cyst. I had it removed in 2005. It was the surgery that caused the injury,' he turns to me, 'right?'

'Yes.'

'And it affects your memory?' says Joe.

'Yes, quite badly. And sometimes my behaviour. I have fatigue also, quite badly.'

'God.'

Joe looks concerned. Like so many people we meet, this may be the first time he has heard of anything like this – the idea that you might acquire a disability from a life-saving operation, that amnesia might be a real thing, something you might have to live with, not just something you hear about in films.

'Ah,' says Matthew, 'there are worse things.'

The route from the camping field to the Hendrick's area leads us behind the main stage at a distance of about a hundred feet.

'Oh, man,' says Matthew, 'that's not good.' He raises a hand to his good ear. Back here the music sounds dreadful – just a woolly racket that pulses through the body unpleasantly.

'It's because the bass travels in waves which are lo-ong,' says Matthew, 'they are more stable and can get through everything. The higher sounds have short little waves and get messed up. The further away you get from the source of the noise, the more you just hear the bass.'

Back at the Hendrick's tent we are approached by a lady in tweed plus-fours who engages us in a stagy conversation about what wonders we have seen today and whether we have made a contribution to the Hendrick's Carnival of Knowledge. She offers us each a slip of paper and a short pencil, explaining that we can write down something we are interested in, something we know about that others might find fascinating. Matthew writes, *What is the order of the planets? Mercury, Venus, Earth, Mars, Jupiter, Saturn, Uranus, Neptune, Pluto.*

Perry, who is running our event, arrives with his girlfriend, Claire, and they start moving their gear to the camping field. Matthew and I make our way back across the festival site, past the main stage and the dance tent and the food stalls. Matthew buys a little tray of chips and eats them as we walk. We get to the village proper, with its multicoloured houses. It's like a toy town. There's a pink cafe and a yellow corner grocery. There are statues and fountains in little courtyards. I have read that the village was the fantasy of an architect who wanted to recreate the aesthetic of the Mediterranean. It's also where the TV show *The Prisoner* was shot.

We find a way downhill that looks like it might take us to the beach, but it ends at the hotel and a rocky outcrop. As we backtrack we talk more about the Lottery. I tell Matthew I think it's a covert tax on the poor – a way of tricking money out of people who can't afford it and then spending it on things that should be paid for by taxing rich people. He seems taken with the idea. 'Oh, man, that's so clever!'

'It's a way of smuggling market competition into public services as well,' I say. 'You cut spending on the statutory sector and set up a big fund and make charities compete for it in order to supply the services the state should offer.'

'It's completely capitalist. It's so devious!'

There are festival-goers everywhere, music filling the air, barricades channelling our movements. By the time we get back up the hill, still looking for the beach, Matthew is lagging behind by some distance. I stop and let him catch up. His eyes are puffy. We've been travelling all day. I don't know why he's pressing on. 'You don't have to come,' I say.

'It's OK.' He follows me a little further but then stops again. 'Actually,' he says, 'I'll probably go back. I'm tired.' He almost laughs, as though it's a surprise to him, admitting this.

'Good decision.'

The noise of the festival is like a river swirling around us as we stand there looking at each other. The light is fading and people are staggering and strolling in all directions. Everything smells of grass and earth and beer. Matthew stares at me, vacant, his body sagging, and I see that he has lost it.

Africans don't camp, he said on the train. He went to boarding school; he slept on hard bunks and frequently went hungry. He has memories of catching animals with his friends to supplement the meagre school diet. Why would you do that out of choice? He was joking. He wants to do things like this. He enjoys the contradictions, likes testing himself and other people. That's all fun. But he has a brain injury. He has a disability nobody can see. What is it I expect to gain from bringing him here? What am I doing?

I walk back with him to the camping field and make sure he finds his tent. Claire and Perry have set up next door and on the way past I ask them to keep an eye out for Matthew.

I walk through the zones of sound again in the dusk, dodging through the crowds until they thin out and disappear. As I get deeper into the woods, the sound is left behind me.

The beach is huge and flat and empty. The music pounds softly in the distance as I get into the water. In total silence, a strong tidal current pulls me west, towards the Atlantic. I swim against it and maintain my position. I stop swimming and drift. I think about the last festival I went to. I remember standing by a stream on the campsite in the dark, pointing my torch into the water, flaring up pale ghosts there. I think about the words my girlfriend, Chris, said to me as I left the house this morning: *Take care of yourself.*

On the way back I run into Matthew. 'I got lost!' he says as we approach one another. 'At the tents. I went to the bathroom and when I came out I had no idea where I was. I just had no idea at all. A lady had to lead me back to the tent.' He seems perkier than before.

He says he is going to buy something for dinner.

'Keep your phone on,' I say over my shoulder.

'OK,' he says. And then from further away, raising his voice over the din, to check he's remembering our rendezvous point: 'Hendrick's, right?'

'Yes!' I shout.

One of the problems with amnesia – at least the kind Matthew has – is that it isn't consistent. It can vary dramatically depending on levels of fatigue and stress, time of day, blood sugar, familiarity of location. And it interacts strongly with both confidence and self-awareness. A degree of cockiness seems to help – if Matthew is on good form his guesses are often right – but too much certainty or unwariness can get him into trouble, especially if he's fatigued or under stress. So it's a gamble. In unfamiliar surroundings he relies, really, on other people; strangers like the lady who led him back to the tent. Who was she? Matthew said something about a psychologist. Do festivals have psychologists? Some sort of well-being officer? Maybe they do these days; maybe they've learned the value. Festivals are inherently disorienting, that's part of the point. But some people stand closer to the edge than others, to the boundary of the woods, need less of a push to stumble into the unknown.

My job is to take risks, though. Calculated ones. The whole point is to give people like Matthew opportunities to aim a little higher, push a little over the line. After a while you get a slow kind of instinct. A feeling in your fingers of how long you should give a person before you start to worry. It's about their dignity, after all. It matters that you trust them. It matters how you think about them. With some people it's no time at all. Sid, for example – I wouldn't let him out of my sight. With some people there's no time limit, really.

After dinner I find Matthew back at the tents pottering around. I ask if he's had his shower.

'I wanted to but it would be too cold walking over.'

'You can keep your clothes on. Just go over there in them and put them back on after you shower.'

'Oh, yes. That's a good idea.'

Later, lying in the dark inside my tent, I worry about whether Matthew will sleep OK but I know there's not much I can do about it.

The music stops in the early hours. I manage a kind of clammy stupor just this side of sleep. At 6 a.m. I am roused by Matthew's voice. The first time he says my name I open my eyes. The second time I know it's real. I pull out an earplug.

'What is it?'

'You might want to use the bathroom before there's a queue.' He's talking to me from a distance of ten feet. He's standing beside his tent, busying himself with something, wide awake.

'OK, thanks.'

We walk down through the deserted festival site. The grass is dewy and littered. The tents and stages are abandoned and shadowed. The only people are the security staff who lean against the folding tables at the checkpoints. Matthew says hello to each of them as we pass.

'Hello there. How's it going? Tired?'

'Yep.'

'Been up all night?'

'Twelve hours.'

'Ah, man, that's tough. You're doing a good job.'

They respond to his overtures with rugged gratitude. One of them makes a joke about us getting him a fry-up.

'Man, that's tough work,' Matthew says to me. 'I used to do that when I worked in security. You really realize that time is relative. Time stretches very far.'

We are hoping for a cup of tea, but the man at the gate to the village tells us nothing is open until nine. We make our way up the hill and around into the woods.

We stroll on the beach a while and look at the strange volcanic rock formations that rise out of the sand. I watch as Matthew lifts his boots, letting the sand run out of them. He tells me about the dust on the moon. 'It's some kind of silicate. It's very sharp. You don't want it in your clothes.'

As we make our way back up the path to the festival site, Matthew asks after Sid again. I say I haven't heard about him in a while. As far as I know he's fine.

'Why did he leave Headway?'

'It wasn't doing him any good.'

'His memory was really bad.'

'Yeah. I haven't met anyone with a worse memory. He didn't really know where he was. I think maybe there was a time when it was good for him, but eventually he ended up just feeling stressed by it. Somebody visited him at his home and apparently he was much more relaxed there.'

'Makes sense.'

You assume that social contact and engagement is good for people. You assume that getting away from the nursing home would make sense for a man in his forties. But if it takes him thousands of exposures to recognize a place or a person, thousands of exposures to become familiar with something or someone, if it takes him five years to begin to settle and then you move premises, if his cognitive impairments prevent him from engaging in any activity that lasts for more than five minutes, and if that means he never really cultivates what could be called a friendship – if this is the situation then it might well be better to accept that, in this case, the man should stay at home, go for a little walk with someone gentle, smoke another cigarette.

We are walking through the woods again, back towards the village. 'Can we get some food soon?' asks Matthew.

'Yes. Breakfast time, definitely.'

We walk on a little further. I see Matthew frowning and smiling at once, thinking something over. He looks at me: 'It's so clever. It's just a tax on the plebs!'

After breakfast Matthew and I walk down to the hotel on the coastline and sit in the lobby there. We spend an hour or two reading, and run through our plans for the talk we're going to give.

On the way back we stop at the food stalls.

'How's that guy,' asks Matthew, 'Sid?'

'He's all right, I think. You asked me already.'

'OK.'

Perry is setting up the tent where we're going to be talking.

There is some faffing with lights. We start ten minutes late, but there's a good-sized audience – around twenty – filling the tent. I tell them they should have each found a piece of paper and a pen on their seats. I ask them to write down an early memory. Nothing special, just something they remember from childhood.

And then Matthew appears and we start to talk. There are lights in our faces and people are looking at us and listening and it's all making a weird kind of sense.

For a person with a prefrontal cortical injury Matthew is extraordinarily good at winging it. The way it works is this: I interview him about the things the audience need to hear and fill in the gaps; I keep a handle on the structure and timing so that Matthew can be himself – funny and insightful and vulnerable and razor-sharp.

The last time we spoke to the public was at a pop-up restaurant in an underground bunker in Dalston. It was a 'brain banquet': a neuroscience-themed meal accompanied by talks on curious topics from psychology and brain research. Something like a nineteenth-century salon but with paying guests, mostly young working people with an appetite for the macabre – out for fun, for gore, for a laugh. The main course was calves' brains. The lighting was dim. Some of the speakers had trouble being heard over the squeals of disgust as the food was served.

As the dessert arrived (cheesecake) and Matthew and I stood up to deliver our part of the evening, I worried that the rowdier elements of the audience weren't going to shut up – that Matthew would have his confidence knocked or that what we were offering was at odds with people's expectations.

How do you tell a story about so much loss, about disability, about catastrophic misfortune, about one of the hardest things a person can live through, a story that challenges people's beliefs about the nature of personhood, about fate, about identity – how do you tell that story in a way that doesn't frighten people? Or worse, make them feel like they're being taught a lesson? The worst outcome – worse than anything – would be for people to feel they owe Matthew their pity.

What we need to do, Matthew and I, is explain how he developed a life-threatening brain disease, how he underwent surgery that disabled him permanently, how he lost his career and maybe all of his prospects for a fulfilling future, and at the same time show the audience how this is not just interesting and heart-breaking but also maybe in some ways directly pertinent to their own lives – as a means of understanding better what their own minds are doing, and their own terribly, awfully contingent place in an essentially infinite and indifferent universe. And we also, ideally, have to make them laugh.

We disagree onstage as in life. I ask him to talk about the effects of his injury. He brings up disinhibition: the problems he believes he has with his behaviour, with being too blunt. There's an anecdote about a situation at his other voluntary job, where he sits at a reception desk, buzzing people into the offices of a homelessness charity. He explains how one day a lady buzzed and he told her, over the intercom, to come upstairs and she took a while coming up, and then, when she got there, she was upset with him because he hadn't told her to come through the door that led to the stairs. He says that at the time he couldn't see how a person would not understand they should come through a door if they know they must go up the stairs. Surely stairs are always beyond a door, if there's a door involved. And when she arrived at his desk and gave him a hard time he told her to fuck off, or to shove it, or something to that effect.

'Now, as a receptionist,' Matthew says, 'I understand how this would not be ideal.' The audience laugh. It's hard to imagine him telling anyone to fuck off.

I tell the audience I think this incident happened partly because he was bored, depressed, frustrated. And because he didn't really want the job anyway. I say that compared to a lot of people I know, Matthew is not disinhibited. He says we can agree to disagree. People laugh again.

He describes getting lost at the camping field last night. 'I just stood there with no idea where to go.' He says he finds it hard to know how bad his memory problems are.

I say I can tell him. I say he's asked me about Sid several times this weekend and that he's forgotten that I've told him the answer each time. I say that we spoke about Sid early yesterday and since then, because he's been on Matthew's mind, Matthew has asked me about him at intervals every couple of hours. Matthew is looking at me, his expression inscrutable. And then, looking at Matthew, I say into the microphone that I feel like a shit.

'I've never done that to you before, in front of an audience. I'm sorry. It just came out.'

The people laugh. Matthew laughs too. I have no idea what he will say about this later. If he will remember it.

We talk about confabulation. Matthew describes how he discharged himself from rehabilitation after his original surgery, spent a day or two at home and then wrote an email to the hospital, asking why they had sent him home so soon. 'I can assure you, I'm not well at all,' the email had said. The hospital had written back, explaining that he had left of his own free will, against their advice. He talks about when he returned to work and explained to his bosses what had happened. They told him OK, they would do what they could to support him, they valued him as an employee. Matthew went home and, over the weekend, told his friends that he'd been fired.

We gather up the memories the audience members have written down and I read a few aloud.

I remember a big solid chocolate K that was in my Christmas stocking. It didn't smell like any other chocolate I had ever smelt before.

Smashing shards of glass with my younger brother. My hands were covered in blood, his completely intact.

Eating bird food on the way home from the RAF museum. We were in the back of our white Volvo. Then Mum took the bird food off us and gave us Wotsits.

Lying in a cot and my mum hoovering and I swallowed a penny.

Camping for the first time in my grandparents' garden after being told a ghost story before bedtime. I had to be driven home in fear.

I ask who the last one belongs to. A girl in the front row puts up her hand. I ask her to describe the occasion in more detail. She says she can picture the yellow tent in the garden. She remembers getting into the car. She was terrified. 'I think I was holding a teddy maybe.' I ask her to tell me more about the teddy. 'Yes, we had Care Bears.' Was she definitely holding a teddy? 'Yes, I think so,' she says, but she sounds uncertain.

We talk about how memory is constructed, reconstructed. We talk about consolidation and the way we use a mixture of memory traces and subsequent experiences – both first- and second-hand – to renew old memories; how there are always gaps that need filling and we use inference and emotion to do this. How other things – the stories of others, photographs, other memories – come into play. I ask the girl about the teddy again and she's still not sure. I say maybe the next time she tells the story the teddy might seem more real, a more certain part of it – even though we have no idea if it was ever there. Confabulation is similar. It's just that the gaps being filled are bigger.

Matthew explains that it usually happens around things that he's worried about. When he was going back to work he was worried about losing his job. He knew it was a possibility. He didn't remember what had happened in the conversation with his bosses. His mind filled in the gap with what he felt was most likely, what he most feared.

We take questions. It turns out several people in the audience know someone who's had a brain injury. One man has a friend in hospital right now. He says they had been in the air force together. They were on a night out in Brighton a month ago. His friend leapt from the edge of the pier, intending to grab hold of the flagpole that stood nearby. He'd missed and fallen head first on to the rocks. 'He's in an induced coma,' the man explains. 'We visited him a few days ago and a friend put on one of his favourite James Brown tracks. He started tapping his foot. It feels like he's still in there, responding, and we want to believe it, but how can you be sure? We want to know that we can help.'

After the talk, the girl who wrote about being frightened by a ghost story approaches us with a boy who turns out to be her brother. They tell us their dad was in a car crash when they were younger. Another lady says she was in an accident when she was eight years old and doesn't remember anything from before then. We hand out email addresses. We say thanks for coming and goodbye.

Our taxi will be waiting for us up the hill in a few minutes. We gather our things and shake hands with Perry and the others.

At Bangor I eat a sandwich as we wait for the train home and I start to feel less crazy. Matthew eats a banana from his bag and then stands up and says he's going to buy a Lottery ticket. I look out across the tracks and breathe slowly. After fifteen minutes I realize the train is due and there's no sign of Matthew. I stand up and walk towards the exit. I dial his number, but it goes straight to his voicemail. There's nothing blocking the view of the road from the platform; I can see all the way down in two directions. And there's Matthew, making his way up the hill. He gives a little wave.

'Oh, dude,' he says as he approaches, 'by the way, don't tell anyone else this.'

For a moment I think he's talking about what I said in the Hendrick's tent – about his memory. I humiliated him, made him look stupid. I'm ready to accept his anger, but he's talking about something else:

'The Lottery. Don't spoil anyone else's hopes.' He smiles. 'Blair was so clever. It's amazing.'

Waiting for an interchange at Crewe, we are joined by Jay Rayner. He looks exactly like his picture in the newspaper. I can see a festival entrance band around his wrist. He explains that he was supposed to be speaking at the festival too but never made it because the car never came to pick him up from the station. Eventually he got fed up with waiting. He's on his way home. He asks us what we were doing. He says he's always thought it was funny how the one treatment the ancients used for brain damage turned out to be the right one. 'Trepanning,' he says, 'you know, for brain haemorrhage.'

Trepanning means drilling a hole in the skull. The remains of some prehistoric humans have been found with man-made holes in their skulls. Nobody really knows why they were made.

'Well . . .' I say, 'sort of.'

'Is that bullshit, then?'

'The thing is, unless you know where the bleed is, then drilling a hole is just making more trouble. You could be drilling a lot of holes just to find it.'

'That's good to know. I was thinking of using it in an article – but I won't now!'

On the train Matthew tries to read his book. He sleeps with his head against the window frame, the book still open in front of him. He wakes up as new people get on at a station. A few moments pass.

'I wish we could fall asleep without losing consciousness,' Matthew says. 'That would be very useful.'

'How do you mean?' I ask.

'Sleep is just a sorting out of mental experience. I mean, how useful it is and what it's for I don't know. If you could still be awake that would be better.' He leans forward and rests his head against the window frame again, closing his eyes tightly. I watch him. His eyes open a little.

'What are you doing?' I ask.

'I'm sleeping.'

★

For the first month after fertilization, the cells of the human zygote divide and multiply their number. When a critical mass is achieved, a chemical signal slows the frenzy to a simmer. Up until now the form has been a softly pullulating sphere, but at something like five weeks of development the symmetry is broken, as a disc forms towards the upper end of the bubble. A streak gently appears along the top surface of this disc, a groove that for the first time distinguishes the being's orientation: it now has a front and a back, a top and a bottom. Along the groove, the cells sink, spread outwards and settle into three primordial layers: ectoderm, mesoderm, endoderm. The embryo is still smaller than a daisy petal but, these three layers in place, it now has the raw materials to form all the tissues in the adult body.

The bottom layer will form gradually into the respiratory and digestive tracts of the infant. The middle layer will eventually differentiate into all the internal tissues of the body: bone, blood, muscle, connective tissue. The top layer will form what's left, including the nervous system.

It is sometime during this process of stratification that a colloid cyst will appear. In Matthew's case, this was happening during the early part of November 1977. He had no vascular system to speak of. His limbs were not yet grown. His heart was an unbeating knot. His whole body was no bigger than a pip.

Given the cellular origami taking place, it is perhaps appreciable how some of these evolving tissues might become misplaced or intermixed. Nevertheless, the facts seem infinitely strange to me: a fragment of the innermost cell layer, the endoderm, somehow migrates to the tip of the neural tube – the line of ectodermal cells that have sunk into the body in order to form the nervous system. As the cells assume their mature forms, the fugitives reveal themselves as a pearl of epithelium – of mucus membrane intended for the lungs – sealed now at the very heart of the foetus's central nervous system, in a fluid-filled cavity surrounded by the two large hemispheres of the brain, themselves enclosed beneath the hardening dome of the skull.

At the time of Matthew's birth I was six weeks old, living in a cottage in Somerset with my parents and my older brother, with sawdust on the flagstones. My stepmother, Meg, was thirty-four years old, living in Mid Wales, working in wild bird conservation. None of us had met her yet. She was beautiful, pale-skinned, determined. She too was carrying fate's secrets inside the black cave of her brain – if only there had been some way to see them.

My friend Danny was two years old, a rudely healthy toddler who would look adults squarely in the eye and could already tell when people were talking about him.

Liah, who I would not meet for many years, was yet to be born. The virus that would change her life was in her young mother's blood, or in the blood of the man that would pass it to her, or the blood of the woman or man that would pass it to him.

2016

Friday 12 February.

'So in this one you can see there's an absolutely massive haematoma.'

The brain appears as a clean oval of grey in a screen as black as the night outside the office. The skull is a ring of pure white.

My aunt Juliet recently retired from her career as a neuroradiologist. She's kindly agreed to talk me through some particularly important scans. They were taken just under six years ago, on 14 and 15 May 2010. I know the dates because I wrote about them in my diary at the time. It's taken me this long to feel all right about looking at them – to feel like it's allowed.

Juliet scrolls through the images quietly for a moment, back and forth, creating a moving picture that runs down through the inside of the head from top to bottom.

'You have to try to visualize it in three dimensions,' she says. 'It gets easier with experience.'

Juliet has spent thirty years helping surgeons and neurologists interpret these kinds of images. Despite her repeated reminders that she's retired, and therefore not technically qualified to offer a clinical opinion, there can't be many people more senior in the field.

Sometimes when you sit with a person of great skill you get a strange kind of energy from them. I can almost feel the hidden thing Juliet is doing: building that three-dimensional object in her mind, reconstructing the events of a wordless history.

'There's bleeding into the right temporal lobe,' she says, looking at the first set of scans, taken just before midnight on 14 May. The haematoma is not difficult to see: an enormous patch of speckled white that has eaten in from the side.

With a stroke, as with Matthew's cyst, the big problem is pressure. But here it's blood taking up the space rather than water. Juliet points

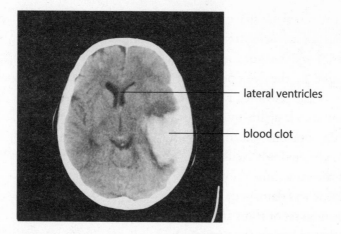

out how in the scans the two lateral ventricles, normally symmetrical like the pips in an apple, are beginning to pinch and deform as they are squeezed sideways by the blood and the brain tissue it has displaced.

'And then the blood has ruptured into the lateral ventricle and gone down through the foramen of Monro.' She points at a little bright streak in the grey: 'There.'

The blood has forced its way into the uppermost of the water cavities in the brain and then travelled down the little passage that connects it with the third ventricle, the one in the middle – the same chamber that houses Matthew's cyst.

It's difficult to think about a person's own blood, the very fluid of her life, wreaking such havoc inside the soft tissue of her brain. It's hard to tell how Juliet feels about it. But she's a professional at this, I remind myself.

'I can tell you Meg wasn't bleeding at the time these first scans were being done.' Juliet explains that in a big haemorrhage like this there is no way for a surgeon to stop the bleeding. If it hasn't stopped of its own accord the person will die before they get to hospital. So what we're seeing in these scans was already old news: the traces of a catastrophe whose principal cause was already resolved. All the surgeons could hope for was damage limitation.

We open the next set of scans, taken the following day, 15 May.

'OK,' says Juliet, 'somebody's put some air in her head now.' She points at the black spaces where the brain has retreated a little from the walls of its enclosure. 'I didn't realize they'd operated.'

'Yes,' I say, 'we got there after it was done.'

'Right. So they've opened her head and removed the haematoma to relieve the pressure. That's where the air has come from.'

I am struck again by the audacity of brain surgery – the act of opening someone's head, exposing their brain to air and light, the organ, perplexingly, with which they see, hear and feel the world.

'At the same time they'll have taken out part of the temporal lobe because it was damaged,' says Juliet.

The next set of scans are from a CT angiogram taken earlier on the same day, showing the cerebral blood vessels lit up by a radioactive dye injected into the circulation – another kind of contrast agent.

'They were looking to see if there's an aneurysm on any of the arteries,' Juliet explains, 'that could have ruptured and caused the bleed. I can see displaced blood vessels around the bleed, but I'm not seeing any prominent vessels going to it,' she continues, 'which suggests it wasn't an aneurysm.'

She scrolls down a little further, reaching the point about halfway down the inside of the head, and pauses.

'Oh dear,' she says, 'this is nasty. Do you see that? That's the cerebellum. It's swollen right up. The whole thing is infarcted.' She points out the dull area at the rear of the brain, where the tissue has died.

She scrolls down again. 'She's got the same thing in her posterior cerebral artery region as well. And the whole of the right middle cerebral artery territory has infarcted. The arteries have gone into spasm, cutting off the blood supply.'

'Spasm is very hard to reverse,' she says. 'And that's often what people die of in stroke – infarct.'

Juliet pauses on one image taken at the very centre of the head.

'I can see now what's happened,' she says. In the middle of the image is a bright ring of vessels about an inch across. 'That's the circle of Willis.'

She explains that the circle of Willis is a crown of arteries right at the beginning of the cerebral blood supply. The circle connects all the major arteries together before they branch out to the various lobes of

the brain. The circle is a kind of fail-safe mechanism in the blood supply. If something goes wrong with one artery, the circle acts as a way
of bypassing the problem – siphoning blood from the other vessels
in order to keep the affected part of the brain supplied.

'But you see it's variable,' says Juliet. 'Not everybody has a complete circle.'

Juliet points to the left side of the scan where, clearly visible, is a
break in the ring – a section of this circle that simply never grew.

'So when her vessels went into spasm and her circulation blocked off
on the right,' says Juliet, 'there was no other way for the blood to go.'

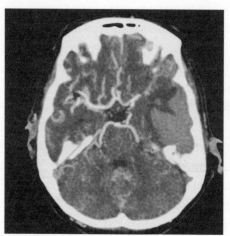 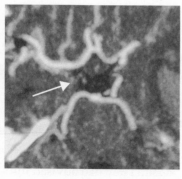

★

I can faintly remember sitting on the train that morning in May,
looking at the mirror-like tributaries of the Thames that snake about
the railway just outside London – the reeds and birches standing in
wet-rooted flanks, and the patches of the sky that flash up at you
from the darkness between them – but I'm sure this is reconstruction,
confabulation from the many times I've made that journey.

What I do remember clearly is the phone call, and the sudden emptiness I felt afterwards – the halt it brought my mind to, like a red
signal shining, silent and implacable.

'Ben,' my dad's voice said, calmly. 'It's Meg.' He was always polite, my dad, almost never emotional. But as he said it, said the words 'she's had a stroke', his voice caught in his throat. It's hard to forget that sound. Or the fact that immediately afterwards he apologized, as though allowing himself to communicate his strong feelings about his wife's sudden illness was something to be sorry for.

He explained that Meg's friend Annie had found her the previous afternoon, lying on the floor of her house in Axbridge. Annie had called an ambulance and gone with Meg to the nearest A&E department, at Weston General Hospital in Weston-super-Mare. Annie had been under the impression that the hospital had phoned Dad. She'd rung to check the following morning and found out he hadn't heard. She'd said she was sorry. That was about an hour ago.

Dad had called the hospital. Yes, they had said, Meg had spent the preceding afternoon with them but had been transferred last night to the neurosurgical unit at Frenchay Hospital, just outside Bristol. Dad had called Frenchay. They explained that Meg had been in a coma upon arrival. The scans had shown a large bleed. They had operated to remove the worst of the clot. She was still under anaesthetic. They would withdraw the anaesthetic during the day and see what happened. They had advised him to come in.

'It doesn't sound good,' said my dad.

'There's no way of telling yet,' I said, 'we'll just have to go and see.'

My train would pass through Bristol. Dad agreed to meet me at the station. We hung up.

I looked at the time: 11.30 a.m. If there were no delays then by 1 p.m. Dad and I would be at Meg's bedside. But she'd been found the day before – Dad had said at around 2 p.m. – and she'd been lying there on the landing for some time before that. Even at the most conservative estimate it was already at least twenty-two hours since her stroke. And I knew that in those twenty-two hours irreversible decisions had already been made.

I don't know how I spent the remainder of the journey. I imagine I probably texted my brother, John. I know I wrote a few things in my diary, trying to pin down my thoughts. I remember somehow the same few sentences kept echoing in my mind. *Meg is comatose. She is alive. And we are already too late.*

I knew that her future, and ours, had in all likelihood already been set.

When they separated in 2004, Dad and Meg had been married for twenty years. Dad had continued to live in the cottage he'd reno-vated decades earlier, Meg having moved to Axbridge, a few miles north. They were closer now in many ways than when they'd lived together. I remember watching them holding each other and smiling now, finally, without expectations. They saw each other every few days and talked regularly on the phone. But my dad certainly would not have known anything had happened to Meg had it not been for Annie. Had it not been for Annie, Meg would surely have died there on her carpet at the top of her stairs.

Frenchay Hospital was a maze of single-storey wartime barracks and post-war prefabs interconnected by miles of identical corridor in a layout that lacked any discernible plan. Finding the neurosurgical ward seemed to take for ever, my elderly dad struggling along those interminable vinyl-floored walkways with his stick. I remember there seemed to be nobody else around. I remember trying to stop myself elaborating on any particular line of thinking, on the ideas that had turned around in my head on the train ride. I focused instead on Dad, on the weave of his feet and stick, on getting him there.

When we finally found her, Meg was in a screened-off corner of a quiet ward. There was sunlight at the large window beside her bed. Everything was pale blue except her. She was pink and yellow and brown. A breathing tube obscured her mouth. Her eyes were closed, her pale lashes blending into her skin. Her fine blonde hair seemed to have almost vanished, as though it might have fallen out, and a white dressing covered part of the side of her head. She was silent. Her breathing, controlled by the machine next to the bed, was as steady as a metronome.

Dad stood and leaned on his stick and watched her. I couldn't tell what he was feeling or thinking. He looked defenceless, tired.

I remember a complex set of uncomfortable feelings, looking at

Meg. Fear, disgust, shame. She seemed exposed in a way that was hard to tolerate, her body too vulnerable, as though I might damage her further if I approached. But I also felt I was offending against her privacy suddenly. Without thinking I had crossed a boundary and was trespassing on her inner life. And there was a further, simpler dissonance. I had never looked after Meg directly – never been her carer in the way I had with my dad. We had never acquired that kind of intimacy. Her condition now, and my witnessing of it, was incompatible with the relationship I had, until this moment, had with her.

I fought the urge to leave. I knew I had to stay with Dad, to make some kind of effort. And then I asked myself, what if Meg can hear us? I didn't believe it was possible – but how could I know? I couldn't just leave without saying something, without trying to make contact, just in case. I forced myself to reach out and touch Meg's forearm. It felt as I remembered – her skin had always been very soft. She didn't move.

Dad put his hand on hers. She didn't move. Her fingers didn't flex or try to grasp his. After a moment Dad said something to her, quietly. He nodded his head and stroked her arm. He took his hand away and she didn't move.

We sat in a small office while a doctor explained what had happened, what the plan was.

Clinicians know that most members of the public conflate coma with sleep: something from which their loved one will, at some point, wake up. How can you blame them? This is how it is presented in the press, in films and soap operas, in TV news. To the innocent eye, coma looks just like sleep.

I am not a clinician; I have no medical training. What I know comes from having spent time with people who have survived brain injuries and with health professionals – the therapists who work at Headway, the consultants who periodically check up on our members. But I know that coma and sleep are nothing like each other. I know that sleep is the rest cycle of the healthy nervous system, full of purposeful brain activity, full of life. I know that, by contrast, coma is caused by a derailment of the brain processes that keep a person sensate. A stroke or other injury switches a person off the way a computer is switched off if you pull the plug or drop it from a first-floor window.

I know a comatose person cannot be roused – by their name, by a light shining in their eye, by a pinch to the arm or a slap to the face. So unlike sleep is coma that one of its defining characteristics is that patients in coma do not have a sleep cycle. They are no more asleep than they are awake.

How should a doctor explain this to someone who has just found out their wife/mother/son has had a stroke? A car accident? A heart attack that, though it has not killed them, might yet leave them with irreversible neurological damage? The doctor doesn't want to give family members false hope: they must absolutely know that to recover from coma is nothing like waking up from sleep; they must somehow be informed that their loved one may never be the same again. But how, at a time like this, should the doctor begin to help someone understand the difference?

We didn't put Meg's surgeon on the spot. We didn't ask him for more hope than he offered. He told us they were maintaining Meg's anaesthetic until they could take the breathing tube out. He said he thought this should happen later the same day. After that they would withdraw the anaesthetic slowly and test Meg's responses at intervals as it wore off. With luck we would see some signs of recovery the next day, as she came round. But, he warned, there was no way of knowing what, if anything, recovery would mean in Meg's case.

Meg was still breathing in the same steady way as we said goodbye to her.

★

Brains, like other organs, vary across the population – in size and organization – but I understand that the gross structure is more or less consistent, with certain areas typically holding responsibility for one or other type of activity. So, variation notwithstanding, the functional consequences of strokes in different brain areas are predictable.

I know people who've survived large, destructive haemorrhages in the middle of the brain – at the very beginnings of the cerebral arterial system, where the vessels form a crown around the top of the brainstem. Damage here threatens many fundamental systems and can cause ataxia (loss of control of body movements), loss of sensation, twitchy eyes, incontinence, dysarthria (loss of control of speech) or dysphagia (difficulty or discomfort in swallowing). But in my experience at Headway this is relatively rare, with most strokes occurring inside the bulk of one hemisphere or the other, issuing from somewhere a little further along the arterial branches.

I had speculated on that train journey that if Meg's stroke were left-sided, the outcome would likely be language impairment. She might speak in tongues. She might find no words. She would know what she wanted to say but would live cut adrift from the world. Meg was a writer; she had had four novels published. For her, a left-sided stroke would have been catastrophic.

But now we knew: Meg's had been a right-hemisphere bleed. So that was, in a sense, good news. With either hemisphere affected she might have hemiparesis – the loss of physical function on one side of the body. The cranial nerves cross over on their way down, so a right-sided stroke would affect her left side. She was right-handed, so this was also good, or at least better. But right-sided strokes come with their own losses: comprehension problems; cognitive communication impairments – problems with the way language is given its social meaning, its connection with emotion; difficulties of spatial awareness; and what they call neglect, where the survivor loses perception on one side of their body, their ability to attend to half the world.

As we sat in the car on the way back to Dad's house, I came to the same conclusion I had earlier, before I'd known the reality: if you had to choose a stroke for Meg to survive, then on balance a right-hemisphere one was probably the better of the available options. At least she would be able to speak, to write. And if we were lucky she might still get outside, see the light, feel the air.

Back at the house I sat at the kitchen table while Dad went upstairs for a rest. Dad had been given that table as a wedding gift. It was made of elm. He had painted it with eight coats of varnish, sanding in between each coat. He'd told me that again and again. I could see the marks in the edge where John and I had carved into it as children.

I can remember the first time I saw Meg. I was four. We were in that kitchen. It was dark outside and she came to the door. I think it was raining. The table was there. I remember her smiling, standing in the doorway. 'Hello, how are you? Gosh, it's wet. I've just come to drop something off for your dad.' I don't think she stayed long.

I stood up to make tea. Meg is comatose. Meg is alive. A big bleed. They operated in the night. She is intubated.

Standing at the sink, I heard myself speak a sentence under my breath: 'I don't rate her chances.' What did that mean? I moved away from the words, the guilt at the bad thought behind them. What did I know? Why should I be rating her chances? I knew that her chances – of survival – were good. I knew how good the hospitals were, how well equipped, how doggedly efficient their systems. She had entered death's forest the night before. But the doctors had shone a light through the trees, had gone in and pulled her out. They wouldn't – they couldn't – just let her die now. So she rested somewhere else, in the half-light.

I don't rate her chances. I'd said it on the train – testing myself with it, testing my feelings. I thought about her death but it was a nothing. I thought about her not being there and I was certain: we would take care of Dad. We would do whatever he needed. I hated my thoughts, felt bad for Meg, for thinking her dead.

But the thought was still there, the knowledge that it didn't matter now. Because even if death was an unlikely outcome, I knew how little 'survival' might mean, and how much. I pictured her being fed. I pictured her trying to get down the stairs. I pictured one side of her body soft and loose or bent up with spasticity.

Dad had turned seventy-three that year. About ten years ago his spine had collapsed – the late consequence of a lumbar disc herniated in his twenties – leaving him badly stooped. He had chronic emphysema from forty years of smoking. The relapsing-remitting multiple sclerosis – diagnosed sometime in his late thirties – was a background noise. In the early days the advice had been that he might soon need to use a wheelchair. Though we couldn't have understood it as children, I think the prospect of his early death had hung over the family for a long time, only ebbing slowly as the years passed.

He had lived with a slowly increasing degree of disability for most of his adult life. He relied on a stick if he left the house. When the symptoms were bad he would sit at his kitchen table all day, unable to get going, grey beneath the eyes.

I pictured him walking up the stairs with a tray in one hand, holding the banister with the other. I imagined him trying to help Meg into the shower.

Meg was a healthy person. She had never smoked. Much of her life had been spent outdoors. She had trained as a zoologist. She'd visited the Galapagos. Her small house was filled with books about wildlife. The shelves of her living room were lined with neatly catalogued photo albums, records of her travels – gannets in flight, tropical butterflies – and the bright flowers in her back garden.

After separating from Dad, she had carried on the same way: on the allotment with friends, on long walks every weekend. She was sixty-six years old. She was fit. She was determined to live well and make the most of everything. I dreaded the thought of her returning from the coma – to her new body, her new mind.

★

A few weeks before our trip to Portmeirion, I return home from work to find an email from Matthew:

Hello Ben,

I was at the hospital today. Surgeon has looked at scans and says tumour is definitely growing.
Size by year:
2012: 15.9mm
2014: 16.7mm
2015: 17mm
Surgeon would like to set a date for surgery. Surgeon cannot make plans without my consent. Surgeon would like to see me in 4 weeks.

My immediate thought is to question the facts reported. This is classic confabulation territory. But the following week we talk it over at Headway and Matthew is still convinced.

'The guy I met was in blue scrubs. He was a youngish guy, a surgeon.' There's something in Matthew's manner — a calm intensity — that makes me nervous.

There's only one way to be sure.

The neurosurgery secretary answers the phone brusquely. She is so hurried I feel my heart rate quickening as I listen to her read through the letter under her breath. It hasn't been sent out yet — she's reading from her computer — but she confirms what Matthew is saying. 'Treatment options were discussed but patient wanted time to talk to his family.'

'I'm sorry to be a pain,' I say, 'but we need to be totally clear. What treatment options were discussed?'

'Surgery.'

I have long assumed that the risks of repeat surgery would be similar to those present the first time around and so have tried to convince Matthew that he must forget about the cyst unless and until they tell him it's become a problem. But now exactly that has happened. Somewhere in the silence, behind the blank sheet that veils the workings of the health system, a new position has been assumed. Against the light, the pearl in the centre of Matthew's head has been measured, re-measured, dispassionately appraised. Flow charts have been followed, protocols referred to, updated, checked again.

Matthew's cyst has regrown. A threshold has been reached. The cyst must be removed.

Matthew sits quietly opposite me as I wrestle with these new parameters.

'So, I suppose the techniques have moved on,' I say. 'The chances are they'll do a better job this time, right?'

Matthew's face is grey. 'We'll have to see how it goes.'

'They'll probably be able to do it more carefully, with less damage.'

'Sure.'

'Who knows,' I say, 'maybe you were right all along. Maybe when they take the cyst out your symptoms will improve.'

'Yep,' says Matthew, 'maybe.'

'And at the very least, now you'll be rid of it.'

Matthew says nothing.

A month later I walk into the hospital reception area and look around. It's the same hospital Matthew has been seen by for many years, the same one I met him at for his MRI scan back in August and for the subsequent consultation. But this time there's no sign of Matthew. I ask at the desk and they tell me he's already gone in. Immediately I'm annoyed. They shouldn't start early like this. They of all people should understand the need for patients to have advocates. At the same time I bet Matthew didn't object. I walk quickly down the corridor and draw a breath before I knock on the consulting-room door.

The room beyond is small and grey with no windows. I recognize the consultant. He's not the doctor that Matthew has seen most recently, the younger one who suggested the surgery. This man is older. He has an accent that's hard to identify, receding hair, looks permanently tired, as many consultants seem to. We met a year before at one of Matthew's prior consultations.

Matthew is sitting next to the desk with his back against the wall, notebook open on his lap. He looks at me in a strange, ambiguous way as I pull a chair forward and sit down.

'Where are we?' I ask.

'The cyst has not grown,' Matthew says.

I turn to the consultant. My look of confusion must be obvious.

'That's correct,' he says. 'No growth over the last two years.' He is sitting facing his computer terminal, at a right angle to us. Matthew's brain scan is there on the screen.

'Right,' I say. 'So . . .'

'So we continue to treat it conservatively. No need for any intervention at this time.'

I look at Matthew but he avoids my gaze. Instead he looks at the consultant. 'Can you confirm the measurements of the cyst?' he asks.

'Well, that's not really so important,' says the consultant. 'It's not so easy to measure.'

'Ah, OK,' says Matthew. 'The other doctor, when I saw him last month, he told me the cyst was growing and he gave me the measurements.'

'Well, that's OK,' says the consultant, 'but it's not so relevant. You can't really make measurements like that.' Though he's looking at us, his body is still turned towards the computer on his desk. His fingers are laced and he's resting his hands on the arm of his swivel chair – body language that makes me feel that perhaps he'd rather not be talking to us.

'So,' I begin, 'just to be clear, you're saying that surgery is currently not under consideration.'

'That's correct,' says the consultant. 'We'll continue to treat conservatively for the time being.' He gives a tight smile, nods, but offers no further comment.

'The other doctor seemed to give Matthew the impression that surgery was necessary,' I say.

'Decisions of this kind are made by the multidisciplinary team,' says the consultant, his eyes expressionless. 'My colleague who saw you made a referral to the team and then we made the decision.'

'That's not what happened,' I say. 'I spoke to the secretary. She read the letter from her screen. Matthew was told he needed surgery.'

The consultant is about to speak again when the door opens. It's Matthew's sister, Ayo. It's quarter past four. She's on time but, like me, has been made late by the appointment's early start. She seems flustered. The consultant, Matthew and I are silent as she puts her bag down and pulls up a chair. When Ayo is settled, the consultant, still without turning in his seat, recounts the situation briefly for her.

Ayo is clearly baffled. She looks at us, at the doctor. She clears her throat. She explains that the assertions made at the last meeting had been quite alarming. She says that she had asked the other doctor whether it would be possible for Matthew to travel to see his family before the surgery and that he had advised against this because 'anything could change' in a short period of time. She says that the doctor had given her the impression that the cyst was now a threat to Matthew's life and that surgery was unavoidable.

After a pause, the consultant says, 'The other doctor you saw is junior to me. He isn't supposed to make decisions about surgery like this. The risk associated with repeat surgery is higher than with first-time surgery.'

I ask the consultant to explain the risks. He says that the fact that Matthew's original surgery resulted in memory impairment suggests the surgeon had to cut or stretch part of his brain in order to reach the cyst. This lines up with what Mr Hau told us.

'The fornix?' I ask.

'That's correct,' says the consultant. 'And in the case of repeat surgery, the surgeon would likely have to again cut or damage the same area to reach the cyst because there may have been scarring or healing in that region. So you would be losing any healing that happened there. And this would carry a significant risk of further memory impairment. The same problem again or worse.'

I can't tell if the consultant has considered how confusing this apparent U-turn might be for Matthew and Ayo, or how much stress it might cause them. I can't tell if he is annoyed with his junior colleague for having stepped outside the chain of command. I can't tell if he thinks what has happened is acceptable or if he's privately furious about it. The single, overriding impression I get is that he is saying as little as he feels he can, that he just wants the conversation to be over.

Ayo asks if it's safe for Matthew to travel.

'Travel should be perfectly safe,' the consultant says.

Ayo sits back in her chair, lost for words.

It's only once we're outside the hospital that I realize Matthew hasn't spoken for several minutes. As we move away from the building I'm suddenly aware that I took my eyes off him towards the end of the meeting and have no idea what's going on in his mind.

'What do you think, Matthew?' I ask.

'That guy is so fucking arrogant.'

Ayo and I look at one another. He sounds extremely angry.

'The guy is just pulling rank,' he says. 'The whole thing is bullshit.'

'Wasn't he just trying to cover his arse?' I say.

Matthew stops walking and turns to face me. 'Apologies, Ben, but you don't know what this is like, living like this.'

'Matthew,' Ayo says, 'you're being unreasonable.'

He turns to her and holds up his hand, flat. 'Ayo. You have no idea.' His voice is hard. 'Living with the cyst is impossible. I'm exhausted every single day,' he emphasizes each word, like a hammer striking a nail. 'I cannot carry on like this.'

I've seen him this angry only once before, at work after the filming project fell apart. His anger is terrible because it comes so rarely. It's cold and full of rejection.

And now I realize how far from Matthew's own agenda I had moved during the meeting. I had been distracted by the confusion about the assessment and by trying to read the consultant's behaviour. Meanwhile, what Matthew was hearing was the closing of a door. In our discussion at Headway I'd suggested that the operation might go better this time, that Matthew's symptoms might improve after all, once the cyst was out. But while I'd been clutching at straws, while I didn't really believe any of what I was saying, it was of course exactly what Matthew was holding on to.

'I have to fight every day against the suicidal ideation,' he says. He is a man stuck on a cliff face. The junior doctor's offer to remove the cyst had been a rope thrown down from the top. And now that rope has been whipped away.

'Living like this is no life at all.'

Ayo has to go back to work. I don't know what she thinks as she walks away. I don't know if Matthew has ever said anything like that to her before – about his suicidal thoughts. He and I cross the road and wander up the pavement as the autumn sun drops and our shadows lengthen.

We sit down at a cafe and I ask him about other things in his life, try to gauge his thinking. He tells me his plans for the weekend. He's going on a long bike ride and needs to get to the start point in west London. We talk about films that are out at the moment. We make a plan to see one together next week. I stop short of following Headway's suicidal ideation procedure. You're supposed to check if someone has made plans to kill themselves, and in what degree of detail. You're supposed to ask if they have harmed themselves at any point and if they intend to do so. You're not supposed to leave someone alone if you think they might actually do it. I know Matthew has thought about it before, but somehow I don't believe he meant it was happening now. Somehow I trust that he said it because he was angry, because he wanted Ayo and I to see how disappointed he was feeling, how frustrated, how much he needs something to change.

But later that night I wake in the small hours and lie there with the words 'suicidal ideation' ringing in my ears. I think about him at home on his own and I wonder if he's awake too. I realize I have no idea what he remembers – about the meeting, about anything. And I wonder if this time, in leaving him to go home alone, I've made a mistake I won't be able to reverse.

★

Over the next few months it seems that Matthew's mood takes a turn for the worse. He stops coming to Headway for a while. When he starts again he seems more tired, more closed off than previously. Before the confusion at the hospital, my colleagues had been reporting he was in increasingly good shape – commenting on what a valuable volunteer he'd become these days, how good he was with everyone at the centre, how much his friendships had developed. But as winter arrives he seems to retreat, still getting on with his practical tasks (food prep, clearing tables, washing up) but largely in silence, as though lost in thought. He's polite, as always, diligent, but also terse, mono-syllabic, going through whole days without offering a smile.

I talk to my colleague Anya, an occupational therapist (OT) who used to work for the NHS and has extensive knowledge about statutory services. She suggests a referral to the brain injury team at the National Hospital for Neurology and Neurosurgery at Queen Square. They'll offer a fresh assessment of the scans, a second opinion about the cyst, and might have ideas about Matthew's fatigue. She makes some phone calls and a few weeks later Matthew gets a letter.

★

At home I work my way through the enormous textbook Juliet has lent me – *Osborn's Brain* – and try to learn more about what happened to Meg. I look at diagrams, videos and scores of black-and-white scans freely available online: the softly glowing innards of hundreds of unnamed people. And I slowly piece together the strange, symmetrical, plant-like structure that keeps the brain alive.

I had sensed the strength of Juliet's thinking, the depth of her absorption, as we sat with the images, the way both her mind and body were somehow engaged, despite the fact that outwardly what she was doing relied only on her eyes. It was as though she were softly holding Meg's head in her hands, feeling as well as seeing the movement inside, in real time; the jostle of tissues in the dark.

I want something of this, to be able to understand what happened, as Juliet could, in four dimensions.

Arterial blood, of course, begins at the heart. From my investigations I see that at its point of origin the aorta, the thickest artery in

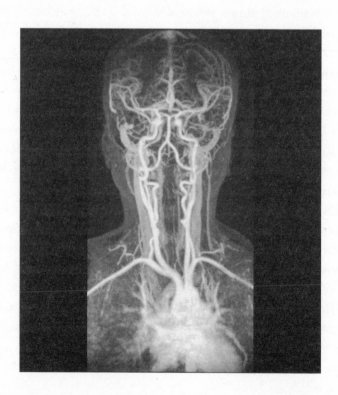

the body, points upwards, towards the top of the chest, and slightly backwards. With an internal diameter that would accommodate your thumb, this is a hose tough enough to carry the full might of the heart's muscular force.

About ten centimetres above the heart the aorta bends double, forming an arch before plunging back down into the darkness of the torso. The crest of this aortic arch, this inverted horseshoe, sits just below your collarbone, behind the top of your sternum. From this prow, the four arteries that supply the brain sprout upwards and ascend into the neck.

Entering the cranium behind the jaw, these arteries unwind symmetrically from the base of the brain. At each branch in the system, the vessels diminish in size until they are hair-like capillaries feeding the uppermost reaches of the cortex.

As far as I can tell, this is essentially a hydraulic system, like the plumbing in your house. As with household pipes, any blood vessel may break if something goes wrong, but it stands to reason that arterial (pressurized) bleeds are more dangerous than veinous ones and that bleeds from big arteries are worse than those from small ones. And the biggest, most pressurized arteries are down there in the basal and temporal regions where they first enter the cranium. You can point to where I'm talking about: just stick your finger in your ear.

Unchecked intracranial pressure forces the brain out of place, squeezing it past the tough membranes that divide the lobes, stripping and pulping tissue as it goes. Meg's brain had begun to herniate in this way – visible in the sideways flattening of her ventricles.

There are processes in the nervous system that modify the heart rate according to circumstance, but evolution has not furnished us with any solution to the problem of brain haemorrhage. As pressure builds, the heart continues to try to do its job: supplying blood to the most vital of organs, even where that blood is itself crushing the organ in question.

At the base of the cranium, the brainstem passes down into the neck through a tapered opening at the bottom of the skull about the diameter of a golf ball: the foramen magnum. With blood and brain bearing down on it from above, the stem can only be crushed ever tighter into this unyielding funnel. This is known as 'coning'. If the bleeding does not stop, the structures in the stem that maintain vital functions are destroyed. And that's when the heart stops.

Meg was at Weston General, the first hospital, for several hours. The team there knew she'd had a bleed and they knew where it was because they'd done a CT scan. They could see that it was intra-cerebral, originating inside the brain tissue itself.

In the hospital notes, Meg is recorded as having pronounced weakness on her left side during that afternoon – a classic stroke symptom – but her score on the Glasgow Coma Scale is recorded as 15, meaning she was awake, oriented and talking. I imagine they were hoping she was out of the woods. I suppose it was possible at this point that the bleed might have stopped, that she might have remained stable, and begun her recovery. It wasn't until that evening, when her coma scale began to drop, that they decided to transfer her to Frenchay. They intubated her and put her in an ambulance. As far as I understand it, this fall in Meg's level of consciousness was the outward sign of the infarct – of the areas of grey death caused by her collapsing arteries.

It's not clear to me if the surgeons at Frenchay noticed the extent of the infarct on the scans and decided to try surgery anyway, or if perhaps they weren't aware of how severe the damage was. Either way, the operation took place in the early hours of 15 May. The surgeons note there was a large clot.

It was later that morning that Dad and I visited. Meg was still intubated, still under anaesthetic. I have no idea what her chances of recovery were at this point. Perhaps, if things had remained stable, she could still have survived. But in the notes made the following day, the 16th, I come across another downward turn in Meg's condition.

I remember bright sun in my dad's garden. I remember being there on my own that day. We had concluded it was best that we didn't all visit. I believe my dad and brother went up that morning. But maybe they missed what happened, or came and went before it occurred. It's not clear what time it happened from the notes, but sometime that day an unnamed person records a sudden spike in Meg's heart rate and blood pressure and a drop in her coma scale from 11 to 6 – a dramatic loss of responsiveness.

Next to these observations, someone has written '? Cushing' in the notes. The Cushing reflex, named after Harvey Cushing, is sometimes seen in head injury patients who are about to die, and is understood as a sign of catastrophically increased pressure inside the skull.

By the following morning, all sedation had been withdrawn, but Meg's coma scale score had dropped to 3 and stayed there.

I look back at Meg's angiogram, at the incomplete circle of Willis.

The original bleed had been big and very destructive on its own, but the infarcts had added a second blow, increasing the reach of the stroke to whole territories that might have been spared if the circle of Willis were complete.

This missing link was a congenital feature of Meg's cerebral blood supply – a bridge that was never built, a gap she lived with from the day she was born, which nobody knew about until it was too late.

Meg was a victim of the same occult chains of causation we all ultimately submit to, the dark iceberg of biological contingency that underlies the sunlit peak we know by day: the outline in the mirror, the dull aches we manage with pills; our coarse and partial sensitivity to the life unwinding inside our own bodies.

Stroke. A stroke of lightning. A stroke of luck – good or ill. The term comes from the days before MRI or CT, before we could take pictures inside the skull and see the mass of white collecting there, when apoplexies were acts of divine vengeance, or might as well have been.

At one of Matthew's neurology appointments some years ago I remember the consultant saying, 'If we could scan everyone in the population tomorrow, there would be a lot of unhappy people.' Most of us live in blissful ignorance. And maybe it's better that way.

★

December 1990, Aiyetoro, Nigeria. The sky is hazy as Matthew sets out. Though it is after noon the air is chilly against his calves. He will be warm soon, though, once they have walked for a while. Hakeem is waiting outside in the grass; they shake hands and then make their way quietly around the dorm and towards the trees until they are far enough from the buildings not to be heard. They find Folu and Dickson by the usual tree, the big one that stands alone. Now there are four of them, enough to catch a bird. Folu has the knife and matches.

The woods are exciting. You could get lost here. You can feel free, as though school did not exist. And thinking about the juicy meat they will cook makes Matthew's mouth water. But you must still concentrate all the while if you don't want to get hurt. Everyone knows about the senior who was bitten by a snake.

'Hey,' says Dickson, holding out his hand, 'can you believe it?' There is a deep purple mark across the palm.

'Mr R?' says Hakeem.

Dickson nods. 'He's crazy!'

Mr Rodrigopulle is the mathematics teacher. He is the strictest teacher in school. Like Matthew, Dickson is not good in mathematics.

'You have to work harder,' says Matthew.

'It doesn't make any difference,' says Dickson. 'Mr R just likes to beat me!'

They laugh because Dickson makes a face, like nothing makes any sense to him. He takes it well; he is reasonable.

Mr R writes a formula on the blackboard and then he turns around and says a boy's name. You stand up and walk to the front and try your best but mostly you get it wrong. Mr R picks up the cane and you hold out your hand.

It doesn't matter if you keep quiet because Mr R is very fair. He works his way around the class and he will get to you eventually. There are fifty boys in the class so it is usually a few weeks between beatings. The problem is that all the teachers give you beatings if you get things wrong. And mathematics isn't Matthew's only area of weakness. The only classes he doesn't get the cane in are home economics and art.

He can feel the sting in his hand and on his backside, like the two are becoming linked by some fiery track inside him.

Somehow, Matthew thinks, despite the beatings, he is still interested in Mr R. He would like to ask him how he came to be in Nigeria, ask him about his home country, Sri Lanka. But, like all the teachers, Mr R is not interested in Matthew. Teachers are rarely interested in pupils, especially pupils like Matthew who are too small for sports as well as being academically uninspired. Sometimes, with some of the teachers, he is sure they don't know who he is.

They have been walking for an hour when Hakeem spots a pair of chickens among the trees. Hakeem and Dickson are best at catching so they go one way while Matthew and Folu go the other to chase the birds towards them.

Before he came to school, Matthew had never killed an animal. He knew also that he had never been truly hungry before now. You start term with a big bag of snacks in your dorm cupboard but that runs out and by the end of term you are relying on what the school gives you at canteen: rice, yam, bean bread, soup. And sometimes a senior will take your food. Matthew is small for his age so he is easy to bully. There are a thousand children at school and every one of them is hungry, none more so than Matthew.

The leaves rustle as he moves. He tries to bring his feet down quietly. Folu is there, a few trees away, moving forward too. Matthew can't see Hakeem and Dickson, but he knows they are waiting to jump out.

When they have caught a chicken they will kill it. They will cut open its belly and take out the guts and cut off the head and cut along the chicken's ribs at the back and spread the bird out flat. They will find two thin sticks which they will push through the chicken's body in the shape of a cross. Then they will light a fire and hold the chicken over it until the feathers are all burned off and there is no blood left and the meat steams when they cut it. They will eat while the woods grow dark around them. And this, like every time, will be the best meal of their lives.

'For one value of y,' says Mr R, 'you have a number of possible values for x.'

Matthew watches the white shapes appearing on the blackboard.

'So, where *a*, *b* and *c* are constants,' continues Mr R, 'then *y* equals *ax* squared plus *bx* plus *c*.'

This is one of the best schools in the country; Matthew did well to get a place. He knows he is lucky to be here and this is partly what makes him unhappy – because he fears he is not deserving of the privilege. His parents are paying a lot of money for him to attend, and he is failing.

The letters on the board give Matthew pain – an almost physical sickness. He wants desperately to understand what Mr R is talking about, but his words move past like sticks in a river, offering nothing for him to grasp.

Every day he is woken at seven to begin learning. He learns to sweep and mop and cut the sharp grass. He learns to fetch water for his seniors and for himself, the twenty-five-litre jerrycan biting into his fingers. He learns to wash his clothes in the stream from the reservoir in the forest. He learns that breakfast is an endless queue in the big hall; that assembly is in the square between the buildings where a thousand heads and two thousand arms riot, cascade, then shuffle in semi-quiet. He learns again and again that classes are from 9 a.m. until 12.30 p.m. and that 1.30 p.m. until 2.30 p.m. is reading period. He learns how to smile and make jokes when the seniors push him around. He learns he is not aggressive. He sees other boys fighting. The noise is terrible, like the breaking of branches against tree trunks, though they are only using their fists. His own body doesn't work that way; if he is going to fight he must do it more slowly, more quietly. He learns to sit with uncertainty and confusion, to hold discomfort close to him, as though it were a friend. And, of course, he learns how to be hungry.

But in lessons Matthew learns nothing. Chemistry, mathematics, agricultural science. These are only words and systems of words, like complex games to which nobody has explained the rules.

It will be several years before he sees what is really going on. As an adult looking back he will finally grasp that even his misunderstanding had been wrong; he had spent all his energy misunderstanding the lessons when what he should have been misunderstanding was the school. At least then he would have been misunderstanding at the right level of description. Because, in truth, the school's purpose had not been that he should understand his lessons, only that he should pass his exams. Sometimes if something feels like a game, that's because it is a game. There were a thousand children. How else was it supposed to work?

★

July 1994, Lagos. The computers hum in the sunlight. Matthew sits and types in the commands. He has been coming to computer college for two weeks now and already he knows there is something important happening to him. He is reading a book at home, a chapter each day, and each day he comes to college understanding more.

A computer has no knowledge, no understanding, and cannot make guesses. It also cannot make mistakes.

It is very sensitive. It notices everything you tell it. It will do only what you tell it to do, perfectly, every time. A misplaced comment, a word used out of context, and the whole thing may collapse. So if you want a computer to do something you must take each task and break it down into the most simple steps possible and then present each one very carefully, with utmost politeness.

It is beautiful to think this way: by building everything from the same-sized components with no shortcuts. Everything you create stays the same, stays where you put it, in position in the chain. You can zip parts of the chain together, collapse them inside an envelope, and you can write on the front of the envelope the task inside. You can stand back and see all of the envelopes together. Some envelopes contain other envelopes. But inside them all, ultimately, is the same thing: clean hard code.

Done like this, slowly, in polite steps that cannot be broken down further, finally, mathematics is beginning to make sense.

★

Friday 4 March. The thing I notice first about Samir Khoury is his hands. They look sensitive, dextrous. His handshake is firm but not overbearing. The skin is dry and clean. They are the kind of hands you want on a neurosurgeon, I think, or on any kind of surgeon.

We are at Queen Square for the consultation Anya booked.

'And since the operation,' says Mr Khoury, 'any problem with vision at all?' He has an unhurried way of speaking and a steady gaze.

'No.'

'And your main problem now is your memory and the fatigue?'

'Yes, the fatigue is persistent,' says Matthew. 'Always there.'

'And how bad is the memory?'

'It's bad. Without the journal and my phone I don't function very well. I can function but I'm just sort of winging it.'

'And how is your walking?'

'No problems with walking.'

'You can walk long distances?'

'Yes, fine.'

'And what about bladder control?'

'That's fine.'

'You don't get up at night to go to the toilet?'

'No. Well, I wouldn't remember. But I don't think so.'

'OK. You live on your own?'

'Yes.'

Mr Khoury brings up Matthew's scans on his computer and shows us the area of the original surgery.

'I can see the surgical track here,' he says, pointing at a faint swirl. He scrolls up and down between a handful of slides and the swirl becomes a pale, worming line following the path taken by Mr Hau from the top of Matthew's brain to where the cyst lay at the centre. It's scarring where, like the bark of a wounded tree, the tissue has closed in around the injury. It's astonishing to be shown this when we've looked so many times at the scans without seeing it.

'Ah, right,' says Matthew. 'I never noticed that before.'

'And you see there's small changes here,' he says, waving at the scan. 'Small scars, I would say, where the surgery was.' This time I can't see what he's referring to.

'Can you clarify where those are?' I ask. 'What part of the brain is that?'

'Well, there are several,' says Mr Khoury, in a way that suggests they are insignificant. He moves on down through the scans until he reaches the cyst. 'There's a small dent here,' he says, pointing at a subtle asymmetry at the front of the cyst. 'They probably tried aspirating it,' he explains. 'Aspiration' is a term we've come across before. It means trying to get rid of the cyst by cutting a hole in it and sucking out its insides. 'They probably found it was stuck, so they couldn't remove it all. It's close to a tiny tract of tissue that I can't show you on the scan very clearly, but it's responsible for memories.'

'The fornix?' I say.

Mr Khoury nods. 'It's one of the recognized complications of this surgery, damage to the fornix. And this will affect your memory. It might affect your energy levels as well.'

Mr Khoury pauses. 'The thing I'm worried about,' he continues, 'is that the cyst is growing.' He puts up a set of slides showing the cyst over successive years. The cyst is visibly larger in the most recent one.

'You're young,' he continues. 'Even though it's growing slowly, most likely you'll end up having a blockage at some point. It can make you blind. If it is a sudden blockage, you can die.' He speaks simply, calmly, despite the terrifying message. 'There are different things we can do. I think doing another surgery, going through this existing track, where you already have an injury, would be too risky. It might end up causing you more memory problems. And the fact that the surgeon the first time couldn't take it out makes it likely that we wouldn't be able to take it out if we tried again.'

'Is that because it's attached to a blood vessel?' Matthew asks.

'It's most likely because of the shape of the fornix, this tiny tract.' Mr Khoury pulls a piece of paper towards him and begins to draw. 'So during the surgery there's a small hole with the fibres going here.' His diagram shows the fibres of the fornix in cross section, passing over the foramen of Monro.

'So when you look through the endoscope, if it's open like this you can take the cyst out. But if everything is close together you'll end up with a small space. Everything is stuck together. You have to peel it very gently and if you peel too much you'll destroy this, the fornix.

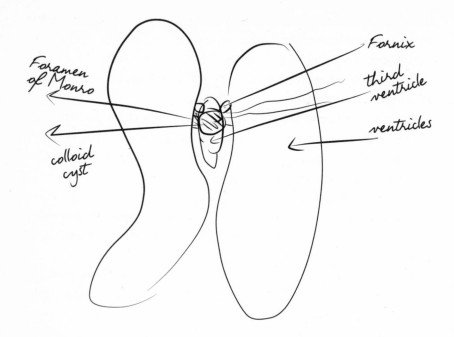

Even a small injury would probably make your memory even worse. So I don't think we should attack the cyst directly. We should divert the fluid from your head to somewhere else. Have you ever heard about shunts?'

'Yes,' says Matthew, 'I've heard about that.'

'Shunts are tubes we put inside the head, inside the space with the fluid, and then tunnelled under the skin to your tummy, diverting the fluid to another place. I think you should have a shunt.'

He explains that there are two ways of doing this: you can implant a shunt into each ventricle separately, one on each side of the head; or you can use an endoscope to make holes in the membrane between the two ventricles, so that just one shunt can drain both. 'The wall between the ventricles is just tissue,' he says. 'It doesn't have a function. So this way you end up with only one tube rather than two.' He explains his preference for this option – fewer cuts, fewer things visible beneath the skin on Matthew's head.

'Right,' says Matthew.

Mr Khoury pauses again. 'There's no magical solution that will have no problems in the future,' he says. 'Shunts can get blocked. And if they fail, you might need more attention. But in my view this would be the safest option.'

'But you would leave the cyst alone?' says Matthew.

'Yes. It will grow very slowly. It will take decades. It should not affect you as such.'

I turn to Matthew. 'What are your thoughts about having a shunt?' We've talked about it before. I know he has doubts.

'It's just the fact that it can fail,' he says, 'and having a foreign body inside you. It's a bizarre idea.'

'It's not a new surgery,' says Mr Khoury. 'It's been done for decades. A lot of kids, newborns, have it and they live with it all of their lives.'

Matthew nods.

'One of your other concerns,' I say to Matthew, 'has been that your current symptoms are caused by ongoing hydrocephalus, or somehow by the fact that the cyst is still there.'

'Yes,' says Matthew.

'I don't think so,' says Mr Khoury. 'You remember I asked you about your walking and your bladder control?'

'Yes?'

'If you had hydrocephalus those would be problems.'

'I see,' says Matthew.

I look at Matthew. 'I know that you have been working on the idea that removing the cyst might improve the symptoms,' I say.

'Perhaps there is rehabilitation that might help you to work around the problems,' says Mr Khoury, 'but with our current knowledge there's little we can do surgically to reverse the damage.' I look at Matthew and wonder if he's hearing this. 'I don't think removing the cyst will make a massive difference,' Mr Khoury continues. 'I think it would be a very risky procedure and will probably make you worse than you are. Probably you have a 90 per cent chance you'd be all right, but a 10 per cent chance of making your memory much worse. I know the fatigue and the memory are the main things bothering you, but the main thing worrying me is that in the future you might have some build-up of fluid which would be dangerous to you.'

Matthew asks how soon Mr Khoury thinks he should have surgery for the shunts.

'I think it's something we should do this year. You don't have to make a decision today, you can have a few weeks to think about it.'

'Just a question,' says Matthew. 'Why are the surgeons at the other hospital much more cautious? They seem to be saying, oh, don't worry, come back in a year.'

'Even in the most recent meeting,' I add, 'the doctor was saying the best thing to do would be to leave it alone.'

'I disagree. We have clear guidelines about this. It's growing, there's no point in waiting.'

It feels as though we are reaching a conclusion. To my mind, Mr Khoury has been very clear. But it seems Matthew isn't yet satisfied, or hasn't grasped some of what's been said.

'I know someone who has a shunt,' he says. 'He said it's completely changed his life.' He's hoping for some good news.

'I don't think it will change your symptoms, I'm afraid,' says Mr Khoury, patiently.

'The fatigue symptoms,' says Matthew, 'or the memory symptoms?'

'Both,' says Mr Khoury. 'The surgery is preventative.'

'Nothing Mr Khoury is saying he can do is going to improve your current symptoms,' I say. 'So we need to pursue other enquiries around that.'

'From my understanding,' says Matthew, 'the memory problem is physiological.'

'It was a complication of the original surgery,' says Mr Khoury.

'And the fatigue?'

'This would be something for a neurologist who specializes in rehabilitation,' says Mr Khoury. 'This is the other referral I will make.'

'It's not something that surgery is going to change,' I say.

After the appointment we find a bench at one end of the small park in the middle of Queen Square. We sit there in the sunshine, encircled by the buildings of the hospital and the various departments of UCL that collaborate with it. The nearby benches are occupied by staff with lanyards, or by patients enjoying the spring air.

I'm struck for a moment by the thought that this is a place of unparalleled importance. We are in the very heart of London, surrounded by many of the greatest cultural and scientific institutions in the world. And what could be more civilized than the offer of free care Matthew has received here? Mr Khoury said he would make a referral to the on-site neuropsychology department for an assessment of Matthew's cognitive function; another to the Hydrocephalus Nurse Specialist, who could answer questions about what it's like living with a shunt; and another to a sleep specialist to investigate Matthew's fatigue. Such a range of astonishing expertise, paid for collectively by the population. It's breathtaking, in a way. And another thought I've had before: it feels precarious, like something we might lose in time. We're so lucky, I think, just to be living now, at this moment in history.

Matthew is clearly occupied by a similar line of thinking. 'There are hospitals everywhere in London,' he says. 'It seems like civilization is just about managing the breakdown of the human condition.'

'What did you think of what he said?' I ask.

'I don't know. I don't like it. The shunts are too risky. I spoke to some guys at Headway and they all had trouble.'

I ask who he's spoken to. 'Ah,' I say when he tells me. I can see why he's spoken to the two men in question: similar to Matthew, they both present well despite severe memory impairments – they're good at covering up their problems – and this can make them unreliable witnesses. They often tell themselves and other people things that make sense but are far from accurate. One of them, Keith, complains every day about being woken up by his young grandchildren – despite the fact that they and their parents moved out years ago. The other, Anders, was recently included in a special focus group at Headway for people with the most severe memory impairments. Out of all of them, he was the only one who remembered nothing from week to week. Not even the fact that he'd attended the group before. Not even a glimmer.

'It's possible that they both remember what happened with their shunts,' I say, 'but it's just as possible that they're misremembering, or thinking about another, unrelated experience.'

'Oh,' says Matthew, 'OK. But all the same I think I'd rather leave it. If I get hydrocephalus again and I die, well, oh well. I think that's better than living with a shunt.'

I don't think he can be serious. What he's really saying, surely, is that he doesn't want brain surgery. And who can blame him.

'What if,' I say, 'what if that's not what happens? What if you don't just die? What if you get hydrocephalus and you pass out and someone gets you to hospital and they do emergency surgery again and you survive but you've got even worse brain damage? What then?'

'Good point,' says Matthew, after a pause.

Over the following week Matthew texts me twice about the shunt. Monday:

> I have been reading up on the bilateral shunts and they sound scary. The failure rate is very high and effects of failure are not too pleasant at all.

Saturday:

> I think I will reject the shunt. The risk it carries just seems too great. All the guys I spoke to at Headway about it seem to have had bad experiences.

It's clear he's forgotten some of the key things we spoke about at the appointment and in the park afterwards. I build a picture in my mind of him scouring the Internet for facts. It's hard to believe he will find anything that will make the decision easier, but I'm sure in his situation I would be doing exactly the same.

Mr Khoury's characterization of the dangers involved in trying to remove the cyst had been subtle. He'd said there was a 90 per cent chance that Matthew would be OK – decent enough odds perhaps – but a 10 per cent chance that the operation would make him 'much worse'. What he's doing here, by implication, is adjusting risk in view of hazard, with reference to the severity of consequence if something does go wrong.

'Much worse' is a fearful territory. Though Matthew's memory is bad, it's nothing like as bad as it could be.

I think about Gretha. After many years attending Headway, Gretha knows where she is and has built an awareness of why she forgets. She recognizes a few people at Headway, the ones she sees most often, but feels disoriented much of the time. She sometimes forgets how to find her way to the art studio from the main centre (a walk of about twenty yards). And she has very little memory of what's happened to her since the illness that caused her amnesia.

Gretha's awareness of what's missing also creates a great deal of anxiety. She talks of how unsafe she feels much of the time, of how she is often afraid of being taken advantage of. If she goes into a shop, will she remember that she's paid the shopkeeper or will they just let her pay over and over again? If she tries to go somewhere alone, will she remember where she is going or become utterly lost? She says she feels most relaxed when she's drawing in the art studio, because the work in front of her connects her to all the moments that have fed into it, all the marks she has made before, telling her where – *when* – she is now.

I think about Sadie – a paediatric nurse before her stroke. By nature she's a competent and self-assured person, but it's taken her years to even begin to adapt to her memory impairment.

One day not long ago I watched her walk out of the kitchen after a morning's work, take off her apron and sit down at one of the tables in the main space. She looked composed, just like a person who's decided to take a rest after a period of work.

I sat down next to her and asked her if she had enjoyed helping make the lunch.

'What?' she said, a frown creasing her brow.

'You were in the kitchen this morning,' I said.

'I never was. I hate cooking.'

'I can show you a video of you helping make the lunch if you like,' I said.

'Go on then!' Her tone was challenging, as though she was certain I couldn't follow through on my offer.

I took out my phone and showed her the short video I'd shot five minutes earlier. Sadie looked at me, aghast. 'I don't believe it!'

Sadie is, after many years and with the help of a closely supportive family, able to enjoy her time at Headway, able to let go of what she forgets to some degree. Like others with memory impairments, she has a preserved ability to retain song lyrics. She's a member of the ladies' choir at Headway, celebrated for her voice and for her sense of humour. But her life, like Gretha's, is profoundly limited. Apart from coming to Headway the two of them have very few opportunities to socialize outside the contact they have with immediate family. They don't have jobs and they rarely have the chance to do anything without close supervision. They each live with huge frustration and with a degree of inherent uncertainty that's hard to imagine, their own histories, their own minds, constantly disappearing behind them – as though the ground beneath their feet were air.

To me, there's really no question: the risk of a worsened memory impairment is far too great a price to pay for having the cyst removed, even if that risk is only 10 per cent. Matthew should have the shunt. But in my replies to his texts I try to be supportive while remaining equivocal about the conclusion. However convincing the case for the shunt may seem to me, I have no right to strong-arm him into it. Matthew must come to his own conclusion. All I can really do is agree.

*

'Me and my friend had been drinking. He decided he wanted to go over to his ex-girlfriend's place and patch things up.'

There are at least two colours in Danny's eyes. There's the

blue-grey background, and there are the fragments of green that cut through it. I can see these facets, like crystal, in the sharp sunlight coming through the window of the cafe. We're just across the canal from Headway in one of the many new places that have opened up in the last few years. There's a bar with chrome taps and a coffee machine. There's some minimalist composition on the sound system – maybe Steve Reich. When I arrived, a few minutes early, the woman at the bar asked if I was here for coffee or for dance; the cafe doubles as a reception for the dance studio next door. If Danny had been there, I think, he'd have made a joke – something cheeky, just this side of rude.

Danny is one of the most charming people I know. His hair is greying these days but he has a youthful energy. His smile is infectious and when he tells a story there's an absorption that draws you in: he looks away, into the memory, and you look at his eyes. It's an animal charisma, a self-possession that some people are just born with.

'I went with him to her place but when we got there, she says no, you can't come in, I've got my boyfriend here. So my mate's going mental at the front door.'

He's telling me about something that happened years ago, before I knew him.

Danny was one of the first people I met when I started working at Headway. I remember sitting with him in the little side room at the old centre with the January sunlight glancing through the high window. Back then his hair was black and gelled. His skin was brown from the sunbed. That was the first time he'd told me his partial story: an account of a life defined by what was missing. He'd said he was a 'naughty boy', he'd mentioned 'bad people' and a 'disagreement'. He'd said in those days he drank too much and was 'cock-sure'. He'd called his injury 'poetic justice'. I don't know what I'd understood from all this at the time.

The odd detail surfaced over the intervening years, usually from other staff rather than from Danny himself. I heard it was a gang of five men who beat him up. I heard he'd been to prison since the injury for possession of cocaine. But for much of the time he and I followed parallel paths within the organization. While I was managing volunteers, he worked on some of Headway's early efforts at communications and PR. While I was making films with Matthew, Danny tried his hand at fundraising. It's only more recently, through the life-stories project, that we've started to work together more closely.

Interviewing Danny, I learned about the intolerance he'd suffered since his injury: being called a 'pisshead' by strangers due to his unsteady walking, being pushed around on public transport. He'd expressed a wish that everyone could live a day with his impairments. 'Not that I'd wish it on anyone,' he'd said. 'But just so that they could understand.'

I also learned in greater depth about the violent pursuits that led to the injury, and about the scale and nature of the criminality that had defined his life before.

It was hard to imagine him in a fight. The movement impairment in his left side was so severe you could forget that side of his body existed. Sometimes I'd seen him looking at the arm in order to move it. Concentrating solely on the stiff, inert limb, he could straighten it at the elbow and slowly turn the hand at the wrist, the fingers uncurling like the petals on a flower. He walked with a limp and couldn't run. He described it as feeling like his left side had been replaced by robotic parts.

His disclosure was cautious. At certain moments he would stop himself, change tack, sometimes openly commenting, 'No, I'd better not. Better leave that alone.' I wasn't entirely sure who or what he was protecting – Headway, to some extent, maybe, from being tarnished by association; or some former ally he might implicate, perhaps? Also himself, of course. I assumed there were things he didn't want on record, that were better left buried. But something else too. I think he was wary of the effect his story might have on the way I felt about him. If he said too much we might lose something between us, something intangible but nonetheless important.

Of course, when you sense that someone is avoiding saying something it can provoke mixed emotions: curiosity, uncertainty, suspicion. But I was never in a hurry to change things between Danny and me. I liked and trusted him and wanted to keep liking and trusting him. So I played along and didn't press him for details.

I've asked him to meet me today because I've resolved to ask the questions I've shied away from before. I've convinced myself that if I'm going to understand who he is now I have to know who he was before. Above all I feel I need to understand the one thing that seems to define his pre-injury life, the one thing I find most alien: the violence. But as I listen I again feel a tremor of uncertainty. Perspective shifts as it has before, as though an illusion is resolving itself, and I feel something inside me twisting, trying to turn away from him, from the brink.

Danny and his friend have been drinking. They have gone to his friend's ex-girlfriend's house. She is with another man. They are standing at the door. His friend is shouting. You almost don't need to ask what happens next.

'This is the terrible thing,' says Danny. 'This is proper violent. And it's me that's leading it. I'm smashing this bloke's head with a hammer.'

It's as though there's nothing between the two moments. His friend is banging on the door and then, with no motion, no intervening action, Danny is hitting the man in the head with a hammer. I try not to picture it. I try to ignore the thing inside me that's screwing itself into a ball. I try not to let my face show disgust or horror.

'Did he have a brain injury?' I ask.

'No, that's the mad thing,' says Danny. 'He had a skull fracture, I think. But he was OK.'

Part of me wants to know more, to be able to picture the attack in greater detail, to watch it like a dance. Part of me wants to know where in the house it took place – the bedroom? The kitchen? And where Danny got the hammer. Part of me wants to know how – at what point – they decided the man had had enough. When he bled? When he fell to the floor? But another part of me wants none of this. It's already enough, too much.

'How many people are there out there,' I ask, slowly, 'people you've done something like that to?'

Danny lets out a breath. 'Ten, maybe,' he says. 'At least that.'

It's a squirming motion, discomfiting and hard to place. It's a little like seeing through a disguise but it's the disguise that's familiar, rather than the stranger beneath. Recognition in reverse. And my mind is fighting what my eyes see. Danny is both a friend and an impostor. And the contradiction is terrible, repulsive. It makes you want to get away.

But, as has happened before, I am reminded that I'm not the only one struggling to make sense of the facts:

'It's disgusting,' Danny says. 'It's pathetic . . .' He looks away, lost for words.

I believe Danny was always unusual. I believe that from a young age he had the rare gift of being present. Unlike so many of us who can't help vanishing into reflection, he was always fully embodied, immersed, alert to the unfolding moment. I think this was why he loved football: the grace of moving skilfully without effort, of simply allowing the body to do as it knew best. He could run down the pitch without stopping, as though the ball were a part of his mind, a spot of light that went where he looked. And you could see the other kids shrink back. They knew they couldn't catch him. They loved him for it – and hated him.

When Danny was nine a new boy moved to his school. He was big and he had black hair and when he took the ball off Danny everybody saw it. Everybody saw it when he scored. At break time Danny ran around the new boy and hit him in the face. It was only half serious. He only wanted to teach the boy a lesson. Football was serious; fighting was just a game.

It was fun, saying the words, making your voice sound like the adults', seeing which of you could do it best. 'What'd you say?' You'd put on the scary face: 'Come here, you cunt!' You'd shout and bare your teeth and swing a fist. 'Woooaarrrrhh!' And then you'd fall over and you'd laugh. Sometimes it would go on a bit longer and somebody would get the hump. Maybe you wouldn't speak to each other for a couple of days but it was all just bollocks really.

School started getting boring: they were expecting him to sit indoors. They were talking about exams, saying how he'd have to study. But it wasn't for him. Football was on the back burner now and he started bunking off. He saw the older kids selling stuff. He found he could keep up with them pretty well. The same things were true in the streets as in football: if you scared people, you'd already won.

A year or two went by and Danny got a bit older, a bit quicker, moved still more easily from one thing to the next, with the laugh. Someone would always call up on Thursday: was he coming out? Everyone would know the plan; it was always the same thing. They had all finished school now and there were loads of them, it felt like a hundred, going out to the clubs. It was chaos. Wherever they went they would take over and nobody could do anything about it because there were too many of them. They would cause havoc, getting as drunk as they could and picking fights. If they got kicked out, the havoc would follow them outside. The police would come and they'd run away and nobody could do anything.

Danny's presence grew with him. His body was bigger and stronger. He had energy to spare. He wore his certainty like a clean shirt and it felt good – the emptiness of the hunting animal. He was having more fun than he'd ever had. He had more money than he needed. Sometimes he would stop and think about it for a moment and it was unbelievable. A boy like him with these big men, making deals. Sometimes he wept with laughter. He was a pig in shit, a fish in the sea. He was taking girls home, a different one every night. He would get home drunk and by morning he was sober, fresh as a daisy. Football? That was out the window.

And then Danny starts to notice things. A fight turns nasty. A friend hesitates at the periphery. Someone gets knocked out and Danny sees the others are scared of getting in trouble. A building catches fire – everyone knows how it happened, a few people say they should just own up. Everyone bottles it, except Danny. That's the secret: no matter how serious it gets, he never takes it seriously. He's beginning to realize: other people are scared, or soft; they feel something that makes them pause. But Danny doesn't feel that way. He just doesn't.

★

Danny is waiting for me at the station. He's wearing a big parka with a furry hood. His son, Harry, is sitting in his pushchair, looking around inquisitively. The last time I saw him he was very new and looked like all newborns look to the untrained eye. Now, only a few months on, I see that he's exactly like his dad: his sharp eyes meet mine with an intense connection, a combination of warmth and curiosity that's surprising in a one-year-old. It's a mature gaze, already powerful, knowing, humorous.

It's a short walk to the housing estate. 'See,' says Danny, 'there's another mess.' He's pointing out the cigarette butts in the chilly kerbside flowerbeds. 'You pay these service charges and you wonder where they're going.'

I laugh. 'It's nice to see you getting stuck into local politics.'

At the house Harry rolls around on the fluffy carpet and I say hello to Danny's girlfriend, Sam, while Danny goes to make me a piece of toast in the kitchen. 'You've done well,' says Sam. 'That's the most he ever does in there.'

'Oi,' calls Danny, 'I can hear you!' Coming back into the living room he says, 'It's true, though. I try cooking but it winds me up!'

We all chat for a while. Danny and Harry play on the floor. 'See? He's already feisty!'

Then Sam and Harry leave the house and Danny and I begin to talk again. He tells me in greater depth about some of the things he did before his injury, adding more lines to the sparse record of his misdeeds.

'This is probably going to sound bad,' he says, 'but when I think about it, I was probably influential in introducing the people I knew to guns. I was involved in some of the early things that made guns more available to them.'

I ask him how much Sam knows about his criminal past. He says he's not sure. 'I think she probably has a sense of it. Maybe not the detail.'

I ask him if there's anyone who knows everything about him, who he can tell everything to. He says no, he doesn't trust anyone, at least not outside his immediate family. He tells me there are plenty of people he's tried to keep things from – people he didn't want to find out about what he's done. It seems like a lonely way to live, but Danny seems sanguine about it.

'In some ways,' I say, 'what's most interesting about your story is that you are these two people. It's not like the old Danny died. In some respects you're still exactly the same person. But in others you're entirely different.'

'On a good day,' Danny says, 'I love the person I've become. When he's good, that person, I wouldn't change him for the world. On my bad days, when all the head injury stuff takes over, the fatigue and forgetfulness and stress, they're horrible things.'

Trouble with managing stress is one of Danny's principle complaints in post-injury life. 'It has a big impact on me,' he says. 'I get stressed out and then it'll have a knock-on effect and I end up thinking about it all the time, it just goes on and on. It's like dominoes. You put them all back up and then something triggers it off and you have to watch them all get knocked over again.'

He describes an occasion recently when a bus driver became impatient with him, cursing him for holding him up. 'I was pleased with the way I dealt with it,' Danny says, 'because I didn't get angry. I just said to him, "I didn't make you stop, that was your decision." When I got off the bus he was still going on but I just gave him that.' Danny waves a hand, dismissively. 'But sometimes I don't do that. Usually once it's gone, it's gone. I just let it all out and then I end up apologizing.'

Of course, Danny's own perception of what's attributable to the brain injury might not align with others'. 'My mum says I'm no different,' he says. 'I was out with her and I said, "Why do people keep looking at me?" She said, "Nothing's changed. You didn't like people looking at you before your injury. You used to go berserk." I said, "No, they're looking at me because I'm disabled." It's because I don't feel like a normal person. I think that's why they're looking.'

The anecdote illustrates how hard it can be to disentangle the old identity from the new. It may be that Danny's troubles are connected to neurological change: injuries to the front of the brain are common after head trauma and often give rise to problems in managing impulses and dampening strong emotions. It's something we often see at Headway. But it's equally possible that he's frustrated simply because his life is difficult. He has many pressures and few outlets for his stress.

'I suppose if you didn't learn ways of managing your impulses before your injury,' I say, 'it might be hard to do afterwards.'

'Some days I feel like I haven't come that far,' says Danny, 'because there are problems that aren't going away, that are just consistently there. In some ways it's got no easier.'

I ask him if he believes in God.

'I do believe there is something. I don't know what.'

'What about fate?' I ask.

'Yeah,' he says. 'Everything happens for a reason. If I hadn't had my head injury I would have been dead or in prison for life for doing something terrible. Some big, serious harm would have come to me. So luckily I got my head injury, in a way of speaking. But unluckily I have all the shit that comes with it. But I would never have become this person if I didn't have the injury. All the bad stuff comes with the package.'

'The things that have happened to you,' I say, 'where do you think responsibility lies? Are you responsible?'

'Yeah, I believe I am. All throughout my life the decisions I've made have had consequences. It was my decision to drink the night I got beat up. I shouldn't have been drinking. It was my decision to go to the club. If I'd made the correct decisions it wouldn't have happened.'

I remember something that struck me deeply the first time he told me his story. He was talking of a time, early in his recovery, when his mother had prevented the hospital staff from withdrawing his life support. 'They were telling her I was brain dead,' he'd said. 'They wanted to take me off the machine and let me die but she wouldn't let them. She said, "I know my son." ' He had become emotional. 'My parents,' he'd said, 'they were the ones. The only ones who were there through thick and thin. But I said to her the other day, "Mum, I love you. I wouldn't change it, what you did." I said, "Now that it's happened, now that I'm alive, I'll suffer it. But if anything like that should ever happen again, switch the machine off." '

It was a potent summary of the dilemma faced by many brain

injury survivors: the urgent awareness that life per se, however precious, is not an unqualified good.

I remind him of this story and ask him if his attitude has changed.

'The only reason that would be different now is because of my son.
Whatever happened I would want to be part of his life. I wouldn't
want him to go through the emotion of not having a dad, even if the
dad he got wouldn't necessarily be the one he wanted.'

But even here there is conflict in Danny's thinking. 'Harry is my
world,' he says. 'He's made me feel so important and worthwhile. Yet
on a bad day I feel inadequate towards him, do you know what I
mean? I feel like less of a person to him. And I worry about the future.
When he gets to that stage when he needs to go to school, what if he
gets bullied because of me? Kids can be horrible. I wouldn't want him
to suffer because of me.'

It seems in this moment that our conversations over the preceding
months and years have all circled a kind of emotional knot. Like an
atom, Danny's identity is a mass of mutually constraining dualities, a
complex of contrary truths that hold him forever in tension. He identifies one only to acknowledge its opposing twin. I don't know how
he manages to keep going in this condition of self-contradiction.
Maybe it's only an exaggeration of what we all live with. Maybe it's
just harder for Danny to ignore or hide. But it seems suddenly that he
might never settle, never rest.

'When I think about you,' I say, 'I have two very different feelings.' I'm not sure where I'm going with this. 'When I think about
the you that I know, then I admire you,' I say. Danny is listening
silently, sitting quite still. 'You're interesting and funny. I always
enjoy talking to you. You're charismatic, you tell a good story. You're
an interesting combination of a bit arrogant and a bit modest. You're
kind of fun to be around.' A strange quickening sensation in my chest
makes me aware that I've started something I didn't mean to: a
thought I might have expressed to someone else, if only to myself,
before sharing it with Danny, to hear it aloud at least once. But it's
too late to turn back now. 'And you're also gentle and thoughtful,' I
say. 'You think hard about other people.' Danny appears to be focused
utterly on my words. It's a rare moment of total calm. 'And then I

think about the stories you've told me about yourself – from before the injury – and I think, I just can't accept you. I can't accept who you were.'

And then, suddenly, there are tears in Danny's eyes.

We aren't born knowing what will come to us; we see only in retrospect those things that had been coming all along, those objects that fall from a great height, right into our hands.

Summer, 1994, Bromley-by-Bow. As Danny describes it, there was no premeditation to the stabbing, no plan or purpose. He wasn't even invited to the christening. It was a mild day and he was passing by the building where the party was happening; people were smoking at the front and someone called him over. He went in and had a drink. Nothing much was happening, people talking, little kids running between their legs. He went outside for some fresh air. Among the smokers a man drew Danny's attention. He was tall and a good bit older than Danny. Dark hair, a slim build like Uncle Shane. He was a bit loud, a bit full of himself. Danny could tell he was from the East End.

Danny moved over. 'Do you know my uncle?' he asked.

'Why?' says the man. 'Who's your uncle?'

'Shane Hicks.'

'Yeah, yeah,' says the man, 'that fuckin' arsehole.'

It took Danny aback. He suddenly felt the drink in him, throbbing in his legs. 'What did you say?' The words came hot.

'Yeah,' says the man, 'fuck him.'

'What you talking like that for?'

And then there's the knife. 'You little flash cunt.' The man is two steps away. 'You can have a bit of this.' Danny has his back to the wall. The other people are statues. The man is on him and there is energy everywhere. Danny dissolves, moves, and the knife is in his own hand. Danny's chest moves forward. There's a glancing motion, round and up. A white shirt against the cheek, the smell of another man. A slap on the back. The man is going down and bodies are moving in, jostling before Danny. Danny's heart is banging in his chest and he's running. There's something hard in his hand – the knife still gripped – so he lets it go, over a fence on to a green. There's no blood. Like magic. And he's gone.

He folded the knife before he threw it; he can feel himself doing it. He takes the police there, but they can't find it. They refuse to believe his story. If you took the knife off him, they say, you would have cuts on your hands. Danny doesn't know how he did it. Did the man look away for a moment? Did someone say his name, distract him? But it happened. He stabbed the guy, this man so much older and more dangerous, and everything disappeared. The knife was swallowed by the earth, the blood by the air. Danny looks at his hands, uninjured, turns them over. He just went for the knife and took it, like it was hanging from a string.

Danny understands now that it's true: he is special.

And now the crime will vanish too. There will be a court case but the man won't show up. Danny will find out later: the man's a drug dealer but he's in a lot of debt. Uncle Shane knows the guy the man is in debt to. So a deal is made: if the guy drops the charges against Danny he can forget about the money. The charges go away. And Danny can feel the energy moving. Whatever he wants, he can take. And everything will come in a rush.

What shocks me about Danny's early life is how little time there was. The period between the day of the stabbing, when Danny was seventeen, and the day he was hospitalized amounts to less than four years.

In 1994 his own vulnerability was invisible to him. If he'd been a longer-sighted or more cautious person he might have sensed the trembling of the horizon, the gap opening up in his future. But Danny never looked further than the moment before him, the shining few seconds ahead. The world he could see – the world he was creating – held no fear, no consequence.

1996. The nineteen-year-old Danny is arrested and taken into custody for another stabbing. He's put in a line of other young men. On the other side of the glass, someone identifies him as the perpetrator. He's sentenced to three years for affray with intent. In prison he protests his innocence. He starts fights with anyone who questions it.

He's put on the bully wing. He's in his cell twenty-three hours a day. He does press-ups on his cell floor.

He gets off the bully wing eventually and tries to keep his head down a bit more. He's in the wood workshop with a friend. There's a Yardie in there. They've seen him around; he's too flash, always calling them 'white-boy this' and 'white-boy that'. They attack the Yardie but he starts frothing at the mouth, having a fit. Danny opens the Yardie's mouth, pulls out his tongue, keeps him from choking. The Yardie's body is jerking, his teeth biting down on Danny's hand.

October 1997. Danny is released early because the prison believe he saved the Yardie's life. He's come out with a good physique after all the exercise and more confidence than ever. He's met some people inside and now he's working for big money. It's like a wave breaking. Everywhere he goes people want to shake his hand.

At Epping Forest Country Club one night he spots one of the boys that he went to prison for. They never came to see him, never gave him anything to say thanks. The boy is in front of him, trying to pretend they're friends, like nothing has happened. Danny slaps him with the back of his hand. The boy tumbles backwards in shock, falls to the floor and scrambles like an insect, panicking, afraid of Danny. Danny is laughing while everybody moves in between him and the boy on the floor. People are buying Danny drinks.

1998. He is top boy. He has money coming out of his ears. He is international. There's nothing and nobody that can stand in his way. He is living the best life he can imagine, a life he knows will last for ever.

With hindsight, Danny's brain injury appears as a ravine being gouged in a glacial landscape, a crevasse towards which he was inexorably moving. Viewed from the perspective of the present, I see him as a tiny figure in the dusk, racing towards the black. Less than four years. It's nothing.

*

The hammer attack. Danny striking the man in the head. It makes me think about Hazel. I met her first in October 2007 when she visited the centre with her social worker. This was at Austin Street, the year before we moved to Kingsland Road. I remember she was dressed in a bomber jacket, jeans and a black baseball cap underneath which her hair was short. She walked with a stick in her left hand; her right-sided weakness was evident, her arm limp at her side.

From the referral documents I knew already that she was nineteen, that her injury had been caused eight months before, when her ex-boyfriend had assaulted her, that on top of the hemiparesis she was also experiencing some language impairments. She smiled broadly and followed me into the little interview room.

I quickly understood the extent of her aphasia when she began talking. She could only muster the simplest, telegraphic verbal phrases, filling in much of the time with gesture and relying heavily on me to guess her meaning. But she was a great actor, and entirely determined to be understood. I was astonished by her energy and her apparent lack of self-pity. She worked tirelessly at her story. So I did the same.

She pointed at herself. 'Working,' she said, and pointed her thumb over her shoulder and tilted her head to one side.

'You were working before your injury?'

She nodded. 'Hair,' she said, and made a scissoring gesture with her hand.

'You worked as a hairdresser?'

She nodded. 'Manager.'

'You managed the business?'

'Yeah!' She smiled, obviously proud.

It was a fascinating game of charades – groping along, alert to the pantomime, slowly pulling the pieces of the story together. But the stakes in this game were too high to contemplate. And there was nothing casual about Hazel's need to be understood. She kept wringing her hands and rolling her eyes with frustration, looking from me to her social worker, pointing, shaking her head if I couldn't grasp her meaning. The incentive on my part was enhanced by the palpable relief she expressed when I got something right.

She described how, on the day of the assault, she had been at work.

'Phone,' she said, holding her hand to her ear in the shape of a receiver. 'Hello?'

'There was a phone call?'

'Yeah. A girl. Hello? What's it?' She tutted and rolled her eyes. 'Oh, shut up.'

'She was saying something annoying?'

Frowning, Hazel spoke into the imaginary phone, 'Who's this?' Then she looked up at me and shook her head.

'You didn't know who it was?'

She nodded. 'Mmm.' She looked at the phone again. 'What? Tiger? I don't know.' She looked at me.

I knew that Tiger was her ex-boyfriend. 'The girl was asking you about Tiger?'

'Yeah!' she said. She looked at the phone again and said, 'Oh, shut up,' and then mimed putting the receiver down. She looked at me.

'You put the phone down on the girl?'

'Yeah,' Hazel said, shrugging. 'I don't know.'

'You didn't know what she wanted.'

'Yeah, no. *Tiger*,' she said.

'She wanted to ask about Tiger.'

'And me.'

'About you and Tiger.'

'Yeah.'

'She was asking about your relationship.'

'Yeah but . . .' She tutted again, frowned, shook her head and said, 'Oh, shut up.' It was a beautifully clear expression of dismissal. It struck me that before her injury, with all her faculties intact, Hazel must have been a formidable speaker.

She explained that the girl had rung her at work more than once, asking again about her and Tiger, but that she'd thought nothing of it. It seemed to me that she still didn't know for sure if there was a connection between this and what happened later, but I could see why she thought there might be.

That night Tiger, the man she had loved, had broken into her house while she was asleep. He'd entered her room and, apparently without discussion or preamble, attacked her with a hammer. The blows had caused a skull fracture and a bleed beneath the bone over the left side of her brain.

'How could you?' she said to me, her disbelief and shock evident even now. 'Tiger, how could you? A hammer!'

'It's a terrible thing to do,' I said.

'How could you?' she said again, shaking her head.

She explained that the situation was still unresolved. 'Police,' she said. 'Hello!' she said, in an exasperated tone of voice, as though no one was listening to her. 'Tiger,' she said, shaking her head. She took her head in her hands. 'Where is he?' She stared at me, fearful.

'You don't know where he is?'

She shook her head.

'He's not in custody?'

She shook her head. 'No.'

'Was he arrested?'

She nodded. 'But . . . ?' she said, her eyebrows knitted with worry. She held her hands in the air, baffled.

'But he was released?'

'Yeah!' She nodded. And then, 'I mean . . . *what?*'

It seemed to me that Hazel hadn't fully processed what had happened, was still disbelieving on some level about Tiger's act of homicidal malice towards her. She expressed nothing but surprise at it even though, as she divulged herself, she knew that Tiger had spent time in prison before their relationship began and was wearing a police tag when they met.

As she explained what had happened since leaving hospital she became tearful. Unable to fully care for herself, she'd had to move home to live with her mother.

I asked her to tell me about her confidence levels before and after the injury. 'On a scale of one to ten,' I said, 'how confident were you before?'

'Ten,' she said.

'And what about now?'

She shook her head. 'Nothing.'

I had been assessing people for a little while before I met Hazel, so I knew it was intrinsically emotional and tiring work, but Hazel was the first person that really got to me. I think it was because she was young. And because she was so obviously in immediate trouble. And because of what I mentioned before: her apparent lack of self-pity.

Sitting at home after work that day, I couldn't shake a terrible sense of foreboding. Hazel was energetic, determined, fiercely engaged in her plans to recover, to see through her troubles and get to a better place. 'Mortgage,' she'd said, talking about her future. 'Work. Kids . . . or whatever.' Simple, mundane aspirations, nothing outlandish. But if I'd learned anything by then, from my three years working with survivors of these terrible injuries, it was that even the simplest hopes might not be within reach.

The chances of her recovering the language functions she'd had before, the functions that would allow her to communicate effectively again with a team of employees, or take a phone call at work, or give her the confidence to go out socially, were, I thought, extremely low. It was eight months since her injury. I knew that recovery could continue after this, but her impairments were profound; there was a limit to what could be hoped for even in the long term. I thought about what we could offer Hazel, what the NHS and social services would do for her, about the intolerance and impatience she would experience at the hands of the wider public. I thought about how long she would live with the consequences of her injury, about what Tiger had taken from her – all the things about herself that she had yet to discover, the opportunities that would now never be known. And I was immobilized by these thoughts.

It seemed impossible that this could happen, that something so monstrous could be allowed. I couldn't, somehow, fit it into my mind. I had never come across anything like it. I wasn't ready. How could a person like Hazel be tasked with living the entirety of her adult life in the shadow of an injury of this kind? How could Tiger, this shadow-man, be so stupid, so terrible, so unthinking, so generous to his destructive impulses? What kind of person was he? Did he not know what he had done, what he was doing at the time?

I've used hammers. I know what they feel like, what they're for. You heft one in your hand and you know what will happen if you swing it. The force is there, latent. The hardness. You grasp it and you no longer feel alone. You possess the world more fully through that shaft. But to use this force against a defenceless person, someone weaker than yourself, someone you have loved? What provocation could explain this? What need could an act like this satisfy?

I tried to think back to the last time I was angry enough to want to hurt someone physically. It seemed infinitely distant. When was it? When I was a child, I think. I could barely remember the sensations involved. Except now I had an echo, a thread linking me to that feeling. For Tiger.

How could you?

★

Perhaps it makes a difference that she was asleep, unable to defend herself. Perhaps it depends where you get hit too – would it be worse from the side than from the front? The skull is thicker at the front, I'm told, more robust. But that Danny's victim escaped without permanent injury is still surprising. It's how the universe works, I suppose. These events are inscrutable. They are controlled by the dark forces of chance, by impulse, by physics we cannot replay.

★

Sometimes it seems to me that there are two Dannys, two distinct beings separated by a moment, by the blank space wrought by the violence of that night in 1998.

It was a simple event, the way Danny describes it. He had a standing dispute with a group of men who were bullying his cousin. He had already chased them down the Mile End Road with a knife on one occasion, so they knew he meant business. It was only a matter of time before he ran into them again. He was out clubbing with a friend. He was taking strong prescription painkillers for an injury he'd sustained the previous week. 'But it was boring being on the lemonades,' he says. 'I had a pint, then another. I was falling-over drunk when I saw the boys I was after.'

He describes a 'heated conversation'. His friend tried to warn him off. ' "They can't do nothing to me," I said.'

Danny has no memory of these events. It has all been constructed from accounts given by others who were there. It's hard to know how much is eyewitness observation, how much hearsay. He says his uncle Shane was there, again by chance, in the queue outside. 'It gets me, that,' he says. 'If it had been fifteen minutes later, if he'd been inside, it wouldn't have happened.'

It wouldn't have happened to Danny? Or it wouldn't have happened that night?

It's clear that the thought of it still hurts his pride, his image of who he was/is. It's another contradiction. 'You would never have thought Danny Muir could get beaten up,' he says, referring to himself, notably, in the third person. A legend in his own lifetime.

By his account it was the cocktail of alcohol and painkillers that made the difference. 'I wasn't supposed to be drinking.'

But, as Danny says himself, he was headed for harm. Sitting in his house that day, he'd told me in simple terms that his combat prowess was mostly front.

'I wasn't a good fighter, I was just a confident fighter. I intimidated people because I always had the upper hand to start with. I used to give people backhanders. They wouldn't retaliate to that because it scared them. I don't know who I thought I was. If you spoke to people from the East End they'd say, "Don't muck about with that geezer," but, in truth, I couldn't have stood there and gone toe-to-toe with anyone. If someone could have half a fight, if there was someone who could look after themselves, they would have beat me up.'

A 'backhander'. It's what he'd done to the man at the country club after he'd got out of prison. If, like me, you're not a fighter, it's hard to understand the significance of this. But thinking about it in context I suddenly understand why it's important, why Danny makes a point of mentioning it.

A blow administered with the back of an open hand has no weight behind it whatsoever. Its force is simply that of an arm swung. It's nearer to a slap than a punch, a blow designed to disarm by frightening and humiliating rather than by injuring. To give someone a backhander is to say to them, and to anyone who witnesses it, 'You can't touch me. I own you.' Only a person utterly convinced of their superiority would use a backhander. Only a person of total physical dominance. Someone who believed that they were invincible.

Danny isn't short but he isn't a giant either. He has a medium build. But none of that mattered. His self-confidence was so great that it could short-circuit reality. He was certain nobody could hurt him, and acted in that certainty. Seeing his actions, others could only assume he knew something they didn't. After all, if a person weren't invincible, why would they behave as though they were? That would be crazy.

So maybe he was too drunk – and affected by the painkillers. Or maybe someone finally hit him back.

★

Wednesday 13 April. Like Mr Khoury, Justin, the Hydrocephalus Nurse Specialist, is helpful, reassuring, clear. Matthew asks a sequence of questions that invite him to go over much of the same ground covered by Mr Khoury. Justin reconfirms the preventative purpose of the shunt; the fact that, yes, the cyst would stay in place and, yes, it would continue to grow. He says that, left alone, the cyst would be unlikely to cause any other kind of problem, assuming a continuation of its current slow rate of growth for thirty or forty years, maybe more. He reiterates the hazard of worsened impairment if an attempt were made to remove it.

But Matthew is persistent. 'From what I've read,' he says, 'depression is one symptom that's often talked about. Also fatigue and concentration problems. And most people that have had their cyst removed say those symptoms completely disappear. Their lives get significantly better. Wouldn't that be preferable to having a shunt?'

'Of course,' says Justin. 'We'd much rather that, but the risks are higher if you tried to remove the cyst. And I think you were saying you experienced some troubles before when they tried to remove it. If you experienced trouble once, there's a high risk you're going to have it a second time.'

'OK, right, fair enough,' says Matthew.

He asks if the cyst can move. Justin says he thinks it's very unlikely.

Matthew explains that he suffers from palpitations. He says it's something he's read about in other colloid cyst patients. 'And a lot of
children have it,' he continues, 'and it's often the heart condition that
does them in, if you'll pardon the expression.'

'From a hydrocephalus perspective,' says Justin, 'I can't see a connection with palpitations. It's not something we commonly see.'

'Is this something you've read on the Internet?' I ask Matthew. He
nods. 'The Internet has a lot of information on it,' I say. 'Maybe it
would be good if you could show me where you've read about the
link between the cyst and heart conditions.'

'It's US-based research,' says Matthew.

'There are a lot of . . . opinions on the Internet,' says Justin, carefully, 'as well as facts.'

'And one person who's had a cyst,' I say, 'and had one outcome –
that's not a study.'

'I know,' says Matthew.

I ask if the shunt surgery involves any risk of neurological damage
itself. Justin says there's always a risk with any kind of brain surgery,
but there shouldn't be any problem if everything goes well. He says
shunts are put in every day at Queen Square. 'The surgeons have
years and years of experience.'

He explains that the main risk with the surgery is infection. 'You
could get a simple skin infection,' he says, 'or something much worse
like meningitis or ventriculitis. But our surgeons have very, very low
infection rates. Better than the national average. We do lots of things
to minimize the risk.'

He talks us through the risks presented by the shunt itself, once it's
inserted. 'The data we have says that on average a shunt will last eight
to ten years without blocking,' he says. 'Some will last weeks, some
will last forty or fifty years. But the data is from shunts that were put
in ten, twenty years ago. The ones we're putting in now are a lot better, so the likelihood is that they'll last longer.'

He tells us what the shunt is made of, how it works, how it can be
adjusted if it's not working properly.

'Do I have hydrocephalus?' It's another question Mr Khoury
answered very clearly just a few weeks ago. It strikes me suddenly

that perhaps Matthew hasn't forgotten. Perhaps instead he's testing, or fishing for a different answer.

On this matter at least, Justin gives marginally more reason for optimism than Mr Khoury had. 'You probably have an element of secondary hydrocephalus,' he says. 'Looking at the scans, your ventricles aren't grossly enlarged but they're maybe slightly bigger than we'd like them to be.'

'Does that have any cognitive effects?' asks Matthew.

'If your pressure is raised as a result,' says Justin, 'then that can cause cognitive difficulties, yes. As long as everything went well, I would hope it would get better. The extent of the improvement is difficult to say. I don't think there's a significant chance that your cognition is going to get dramatically better. But you might see some improvement.'

'And what about fatigue? Could the shunt improve that?'

'It depends what's causing the fatigue,' says Justin. 'I think there would be a chance that it would improve, but I wouldn't say it was a given. And, again, the extent of the improvement is questionable. A very vague answer, I'm afraid.'

Later in the day Matthew texts me, seemingly in a steady state of mind:

> Thanks for coming today.
>
> Will see what is said at next MRI appointment and then can decide from that point.

> Also need new MRI and endocrinology before making a definite decision.

> Very sensible.

But the following week his apparent calm has dissipated:

> Really nervous about this shunt business. It is moving really quite fast without knowing how much there is to gain.
>
> Appointment for neuropsychological assessment has been scheduled.

> Don't worry. Neuropsychology won't affect the decision on shunt – it'll be a checkup to see how your cognition is doing. Should be interesting.

> You seem to think this shunt thing is a good idea?

> I think it's a decision you should think about very carefully. Take your time. There's no hurry.

And in the coming few days his messages become more fearful still. On the morning of 22 April I wake to find this message, sent at just after 3 a.m.:

> Sorry to text you at this early hour.
>
> Not sleeping. Ruminating. I will reject the shunt procedure. Not worth it I don't think. Dying from acute hydrocephalus seems preferable to having a bloody shunt.

It takes me a while to decide how to respond. Eventually I settle on the following:

> I don't want you to die! But I understand it's a horrible thing to decide. Did you get some sleep?

Matthew doesn't respond until the following day, when he starts afresh as though the conversation above had never happened.

> I'm going to reject the shunt. It is too intrusive a process.
>
> I have an MRI scan appointment in June, Neurosurgery clinic in July.
>
> The ventricular shunt is too intrusive for my taste.

I don't know what's going on. Is he forgetting? Or is he just repeating his thoughts in the hope that I'll say something more affirmative? He wants me to say yes, forget the shunt, it's a bad idea. But I can't do that.

> OK no problem Matthew. They said at Queen Square you can transfer your care if you want to. Up to you.

Friday 29 April, 1.11 a.m.:

Sorry to text you so late. Spoke to Ernest this evening and he thinks having the shunt is a good idea. He says that after my original surgery there was debate to instal a shunt but it was not carried out.

Also he says the decision to aspirate the cyst was made because full extraction would have been a 50–50 gamble by the surgeon on my memory. I still rather would have had it out. But shunt here we come or go.

Thank goodness for Ernest, I think. I've met him once or twice; he's a college friend of Matthew's and a lovely person. He's one of the very few other people I know Matthew confides in. But I know Matthew and the situation well enough not to imagine this might be the conclusion. Not yet.

A couple of weeks later he emails me a journal article describing symptoms of psychosis in a colloid cyst patient. The message is in his usual style: no commentary, just a link pasted into an email. I browse the article and write back to him, asking what he makes of it. He says it makes him think his depression may be linked to the cyst.

'I spoke to Ernest,' he writes. 'He told me that my problems with suicidal ideation started while we were studying for A levels. Apparently I have always been a bit of a downer.'

For a moment I think that perhaps Matthew is finally arriving at a clearer view on the origins of his depression, but there is another line at the end: 'It is the cyst me thinks.'

I read the message several times, but I still can't make sense of it.

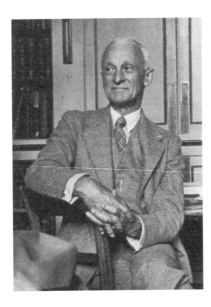

Matthew seems to be saying that his suicidal thoughts predate the cyst's symptoms, that they existed before any sign of hydrocephalus, and yet that the cyst was still somehow causing them.

As I understand it, the cyst is a bubble of gut lining filled with a kind of fatty mucus. It doesn't produce any hormones, doesn't secrete anything to the tissue around it, doesn't interfere or communicate in any way with the conscious structures of the brain. As all the clinicians we have met keep repeating, the only way the cyst acts upon the organ that surrounds it is by causing hydrocephalus.

Mr Hau told us about Harvey Cushing, the father of neurosurgery, precisely to illustrate this point: Cushing lived his whole life with a colloid cyst. Wikipedia says he died of heart disease. There's a picture of him the year before his death looking tanned and lean, his expression full of warmth and intelligence.

The reason he never knew about the cyst was because it didn't grow – and a colloid cyst that remains small and causes no blockage is harmless.

Yet, as though it were the simplest thing in the world, the conclusion Matthew has drawn is that his cyst is making him depressed. Not his awareness of the cyst, not the disability caused by the attempt to remove it, not the lack of employment or prospects he has suffered since the surgery, but the cyst itself.

I go back to the journal article and read it again more carefully. The authors say their patient presented at hospital 'dishevelled, distracted, agitated and whispering to himself'. They say he had 'delusions that people wanted to attack him'. They perform a CT scan and find the cyst there in the third ventricle – but no hydrocephalus.

Some weeks later the poor man is back in hospital with 'a several-week history of a hypo-manic state'. 'He was gregarious,' the authors continue, 'grandiose, over-familiar, over-energetic.'

For some reason they decide the cyst is to blame and convince the man he should have it removed. After this, the authors say the man got better. 'Follow-up four months later revealed no further psychotic or affective symptoms. He reported feeling more settled after the surgery.'

They say they are pleased with the paper because psychotic symptoms haven't been reported before in a colloid cyst patient. They conclude that the connection between such symptoms and the cyst 'remains unclear', but that their case study suggests a link which might encourage surgeons to remove colloid cysts even where there's no hydrocephalus. (I can't imagine what the team at Queen Square would make of this. It strikes me as troubling, given everything that's been said about the dangers of colloid cyst removal. I wonder if the paper says more about its authors' love of surgery than it does about colloid cysts.)

Why has Matthew sent me this article? Why has he sought it out?

I google 'depression as a symptom of colloid cyst'. The top hit is the same article Matthew sent me. After that there are a few more medical journals that report individual case studies vaguely mentioning psychological disturbance and a number of online forums with people sharing personal experiences. Most of them have already had their cysts removed. A lot of them say they had headaches before the surgery; some talk about dramatic blackouts while driving or walking down stairs; one mentions a 'dead numbness' on the side of their head since the operation. One, who has just been diagnosed, says she isn't worried about the upcoming surgery but that she cried about having to have her hair cut. A lot of them express fear and anxiety about their situations, but none seem to attribute it to anything other than the horror of their circumstances.

I can't find anything to support Matthew's theory.

Over the next few days the question turns round in my head. It seems to me that Matthew is morbidly afraid of the cyst itself. He hates the idea of it being inside him and has gradually come to attribute to it everything that is wrong in his life, even those things that could be much more simply and adequately explained by other causes. It's frightening to me. It's counterfactual and is clearly not only influencing Matthew's thinking but his ability to act in his own best interests. Worse, it makes him irrational. And the irrational is unknown territory; it's where people separate, become unreachable. It's where the opportunity to negotiate ends.

And then I see it. The idea that the cyst is the root of his problems represents the one thing he needs more than anything: hope. Because if the cyst is causing his problems, then the problems can be taken away – extracted like a rotten tooth, excised simply and cleanly, forgotten like a bad dream.

It's been suggested that emotions and amnesia interact. I know that Matthew's confabulations are strongly affected by his feelings, that they often take forms influenced by whatever he's anxious about at the time. So it seems probable that the memory problem is not operating in a vacuum when it comes to decision-making about his treatment. He is not forgetting and remembering at random but in accordance with what he needs to be true, regardless of how badly this fits the facts.

The result is a continual round of learning and unlearning. At the hospital appointments the options are laid out, the probabilities and risks are talked through, a conclusion is reached based on the balance of these. Then Matthew goes home and forgets some of what was said. The next day he gets on the Internet and seeks out answers, both forgetting that he already has them and pushing away any that don't fit with the simple solution he desires.

The more of this he does, the more he forgets what's been said to him by the medical professionals in charge of his care. He both forgets and doesn't want to remember. His amnesia is at once a work of cognitive attrition and meaningful, psychic denial.

Conflicting advice only adds to the confusion. Even the subtly different emphases present in the predictions made by Mr Khoury and Justin, the Hydrocephalus Nurse Specialist, create room for uncertainty, for wishful thinking and confabulation. Where Mr Khoury had said there would be no improvement after shunt surgery, Justin had said there might be. Where Mr Khoury had said Matthew had no hydrocephalus, Justin had said he might have some. And I feel the tug of these blank spaces too, knowing that my expertise is as limited, in many senses, as Matthew's own.

It strikes me that in a situation like this, resourcefulness of the kind that comes naturally to Matthew is more a curse than a blessing. It would almost be better if he could just give up, put his fate in the surgeon's hands and stop trying to make a decision for himself.

Is there something I can do to support him better? What would that be?

The neuropsychology assessment takes place in a tiny, airless room in another building on Queen Square. I step out to a cafe while the tests are done, and when I return the psychologist, whose name is Bryan, looks over them and summarizes his findings. He says that Matthew's impairment is primarily at the encoding stage of memory – in his ability to pay attention to what is happening and form it into memory traces that he can then recall. He also explains how this relates to fatigue. 'Everything feels really hard because it requires a lot more effort,' he says. 'It requires really paying attention with the encoding, doing lots of repetitions and associations to make it stick.'

Matthew sits quietly, apparently paying attention but clearly exhausted. I wonder how much of this, if any, he will remember.

'Some of the fatigue could also be underlined by mood problems,' says Bryan. He has tested Matthew for depression and it seems his scores echo his own reports. Bryan highlights the areas that stand out: 'Finding it difficult to wind down, problems with feeling relaxed, finding it difficult to feel positive about life, difficulty work-ing up the initiative to do things . . .'

Matthew sighs. 'I mean,' he says, speaking for the first time in many minutes, 'I do do things, it just takes a huge amount of effort.'

'I think in some ways you're coping really well,' Bryan says care-fully, 'and you're doing all the right things. But it also feels to me like . . . it's not OK. It sounds like it takes its toll, the illness. Living with the injury for so long. Having to deal with the fatigue and the memory problems. It's not pleasant.'

'I wouldn't recommend it,' says Matthew.

Bryan nods. 'And these kinds of things can affect our thinking skills as well because we only have one brain. When we feel worried or anxious it's the same brain doing that as well as everything else. If we've got parts of the brain worried about these other things, even if we're not thinking about them consciously, it's still going to make the whole system inefficient.'

He asks if Matthew has had any treatment for his mood. Matthew explains he was on antidepressants for a while but that they hadn't helped noticeably. He says he also had a referral for talking therapy at one point. In fact this happened as a result of my badgering; it had taken years to get him to try it.

'But I think I'd had enough of it after a few sessions,' Matthew says. I remember the day he told me he'd quit. He'd explained it in terms of the therapist not understanding brain injury. But I'd also felt somehow this was an excuse: in truth Matthew just didn't want to – or couldn't – talk about his problems.

'And are you doing anything active to deal with it now?' asks Bryan.

'I go cycling regularly,' says Matthew.

'That's good. And at Headway you're doing the volunteering, but do you do any group work, discussions or support groups? Anything like that?'

'I have good interactions with all the clients,' says Matthew, seem-ing to miss the point of the question. 'I help out in the kitchen, in the art room. Take people out to water the garden.'

'And does that help? Does that make you feel a bit better about life?'

'No, it's just good within the context,' says Matthew. 'It is what it is.'

After a pause Bryan asks, 'And looking ahead, to the future? What do you want? Where do you see yourself being?'

'I've learned not to do that,' says Matthew.

'It's too difficult?'

'It's not worth the effort.'

I'm used to Matthew saying things like this, but in this little room with Bryan it sounds so much worse. It sounds like what it surely is: an expression of defeat.

'You cannot plan for the future,' Matthew says. 'It's what this has taught me. Just don't bother doing it.'

Unsurprisingly, Bryan says he'd like Matthew to reconsider the possibility of therapy. He says they run groups here in the department, and one-to-one sessions that might help to address emotional changes, and look at fatigue management.

'OK,' says Matthew. 'All right, I'll keep that in mind.'

It's standard practice in the assessment of people with neurological disorders to take a history, to ask where the patient has been educated, what they've studied, to what level and standard. This history-taking is often brief and quite narrow, as it was with Bryan, focusing largely on things like grades, but it's used to construct an estimate of premorbid intelligence, for comparison with present test performance, in order to see what's been lost.

On the basis of Matthew's 2:1 in Maths and Computer Science, it seems Bryan appraised him as a person of average premorbid intelligence. His test results on the day of the assessment were consistent with this: he was, Bryan said, 'within the average range' for most of his intellectual functions. He said this as though it were good news, apparently concluding that Matthew's impairments were not so severe as they might be.

I think about all the astonishing conversations I've had with Matthew over the years, discussions in which he's presented me with new formulations of the functioning of society, economy, culture, the universe. I think about how he's changed since the injury, how he's flourished as a social being at Headway and learned to deal with people of all backgrounds and abilities. He tells me he's learned three new programming languages, gradually, from books. I think about the time we were sitting in the courtyard at the Barbican and he spontaneously wrote out an algorithm for generating the Fibonacci series in my notebook. 'I think it's useful in architecture,' he said, 'and maybe something to do with snail shells.'

It occurs to me that there is an alternative to Bryan's interpretation. Perhaps Matthew is performing averagely despite profound cognitive impairments rather than because of average intelligence. Perhaps, through effort and resourcefulness, he has adapted better than most to terrible misfortune and can, when pushed, still manage a paper exam tolerably well despite what's missing.

I realize it's in the nature of the game: to be tested is to be ranked against others. It's an awful, pernicious trait of contemporary culture: the desire to stream and grade and appraise people for their measurable talents, to tell them what they're good at and what they shouldn't waste their time on. It's not Bryan's fault. He wanted to find a way around it. He was encouraging, downplayed the role of the comparison. And he pointed to something genuinely useful in specifying more closely the nature of Matthew's impairment.

But what can it do for a person in Matthew's position – a person who has lost four jobs since being injured, whose self-esteem has collapsed, whose prior identity was defined almost entirely by their life as an intellectual, who has little save determination left, who yet faces the chance of increased neurological impairment – what can it do for them to be told this? The parts of you that still work are average, OK? So relax.

Just like so many survivors of brain injury, so many people that live with disabilities, Matthew is officially considered a person of no account, an economic zero, a non-contributor. The majority of people don't know he exists. The government would rather he didn't. The rest of us pretend he doesn't. Once a year he's scrutinized by the Job Centre to see if he still deserves the meagre benefits offered by the

Department for Work and Pensions – support he'd rather live without but which makes the difference between a bare-bones existence and begging on the streets.

Because his needs are not 'significant' or 'critical' he will get no further support from the state. Because no one is to blame for his injury there is no insurance to be claimed – as there might be in a car accident – and because his borough has no money, he will never get the funding needed to have proper rehabilitation. If he doesn't get worse, keeps coasting along averagely, that's the best that can be hoped for.

There is so much focus on what brain injury survivors can't do, so much hand-wringing about how expensive they are to support, that almost nobody thinks to ask what they might contribute if a project were made of opening doors instead of closing them.

*

We only have one brain, Bryan said. Even if we're not consciously thinking about our problems, the worries may be running underneath, bringing us down, tiring us out, burning what life we have left in a quiet flame. Poor brain. A hand mirror that holds the world.

An image comes to mind of Matthew sitting across from me in the meeting room at Headway after he quit talking therapy. He held his palms apart in front of him, staring intently into the space between them. 'I like my emotions where they are,' he told me, making that square-sided shape, 'in a box.'

Thinking back over the years I've known him, I realize that Matthew has to some degree been doing the same thing ever since I met him: refusing help, containing himself, drawing a line, finding a way to attribute his problems to something other than the events of his life or the action of his own mind in response to those events. I now remember endless occasions when he would argue that his depression was caused by the cyst, his fatigue was caused by the cyst, unable to accept that either might have an existence in its own right, might even in part be a response of his body to what had happened to him, a symptom of bitter, unconquerable disappointment. He would always get angry with me if I tried to explain anything in terms of psychology. 'My problems are very real,' he would tell me, as though in proposing an explanation at the level of suffering, I was denying the suffering itself.

It seemed to me that Bryan was taking the same position: viewing the depression as a symptom of Matthew's misfortune rather than as some secretion of the cyst. Over the days following the appointment, I begin to recover confidence in these ideas. I realize that it's only in the last few years that I've given up arguing with Matthew about it.

It's strange: if you know someone long enough, you begin to forget whole parts of your friendship. You begin to collude. You come to accept the picture of them they need you to see. To some extent, I suppose, that's what friendship is.

It occurs to me that what we need is some external source of information, something outside the dialogue Matthew and I have had for so long, some concrete record that will answer the questions about his mood and fatigue in a way that neither of us can doubt. Luckily, one such source is readily available. We contact the hospital where Matthew was admitted for his original surgery, and they confirm that his records from that time are still on file. For a small fee they will send us a copy.

Watching Matthew make notes in his journal a few days later, I realize another source of answers has been staring me in the face.

'Matthew,' I say. 'How long have you been keeping that diary?'

★

I have a dream in which there are two versions of Matthew. One is the Matthew of today, with me. The other is a Matthew from the past, in an old jacket, some distance ahead. Together Matthew and I follow his historical twin across a city park, trying to catch up. We walk uphill and see him turn off the road on to a square. As I take the turn I see a small crowd of people ahead, standing in a circle, looking silently inwards at something. The square is utterly still and the light of dusk seems to hover beneath the shop awnings. The people in the circle are not frozen, merely standing still, as though listening. One of them is my girlfriend, Christina. She can't speak to me or look at me. It's too risky. As I look around, I realize both the Matthews have gone.

★

Saturday 21 May.

'Connie eats the lion's meal,' says Alpha to the group around the table.

'Sorry, was that *meal* or *milk*?' says Bryn, to his right.

'Meal.'

I am in a room at the Wellcome Collection, the medical foundation on Euston Road, watching seventeen people playing a game of Telephone, laughing as Alpha announces the result. Alpha had a brain injury a few years ago when he was knocked off his bike on New Year's Day. Next to him is Liah, another Headway member, and then Bryn, who works at Headway as a coordinator, supporting the members every day in their work at the centre. He is both Alpha's and Liah's key worker, so he knows them well. This is one of five group activities we've been commissioned to run today by the museum, helping the public understand more about what it's like to live with a brain injury. Over the last month I've also supported Matthew and Danny to speak here at two small evening events.

Bryn turns to the man on his left, who started the whisper. 'What was the original message?'

The man stands up, smiling, and says, 'Sperm whales are the largest predators.'

The room erupts again in bafflement. It seems the message didn't get past the young woman next to him – who appears to be his partner – without being misheard. She is laughing and putting her face in her hands.

Bryn turns to Liah now and asks her to explain why she chose the game.

Liah sits in her wheelchair, made small by it, and looks around the room. Everyone is quiet now, all eyes on her. Liah is another charismatic person, like Matthew, like Danny and Alpha next to her. Another person I'm glad to know and surely would never have met had it not been for Headway.

She was injured as a teenager by a brain infection that kept her in hospital for many months. And even after leaving hospital she has spent most of the last eight years in rehab and in closely controlled care homes. So now, as she finally emerges into the social world again at twenty-six, her confidence as a speaker is understandably wobbly. It doesn't help that her processing and speech have both been affected by the injury. Her voice sounds soft and fuzzy. For clarity she has learned to over-pronounce, forming each syllable separately. You can hear the concentration it takes.

'Personally,' she says, 'with my injury, I feel like messages pass . . . differently or wouldn't be . . . um, wouldn't be heard properly.' She looks at Bryn uncertainly.

Bryn, a wonderful facilitator, looks back at her and gently replies, 'So, you talked to me about feeling there's a disconnect between the messages coming from your brain – your thoughts – and your body.'

'Yes,' says Liah, turning back to her audience. 'Since my injury it feels like I'm not in the right body. My body doesn't behave the way I tell it to in my mind.'

Liah was studying for her degree at the time she became ill. The first sign of the illness was when she discovered she was losing sensation in the right side of her body. As she describes it, she went to hospital when she found she could no longer pick up a spoon.

She began to understand that something serious was happening when the hospital wouldn't let her go home. She lost weight fast. Nothing the doctors tried was helping. For many weeks Liah was close to death.

Today Liah will focus mostly on the impact of her injury: the ways in which it has interrupted the development of her personal and professional life and compelled her to reassess how she will fulfil her ambitions. Along with Alpha she'll help the people in the room get a little closer to understanding what it's like to lose so much of yourself and still live.

But her extraordinary story predates the discovery of her infection
by many years and begins many thousands of miles away in Eritrea.

Sitting in the little meeting room at Headway, Liah tells me she has
no memories of her father, that she only knows him from photographs. He died in his mid thirties, in 1993, when Liah was an infant.
This was the same year that modern Eritrea came into existence,
finally declaring independence after a decades-long conflict with
Ethiopia, the neighbour that had annexed it after the Second World
War. From what I have read, in the years that followed independence, Eritrea's national politics ossified into a kind of beleaguered
military autocracy. Wikipedia describes contemporary Eritrea as a
'one-party state' with a human rights record that is 'among the worst
in the world'.

Liah remembers the day the police raided her family home. She
was twelve years old, living with her mother in the capital, Asmara.

'It was because of our religion,' she explains. 'We were Jehovah's
Witnesses. We were having a Bible study meeting with about twenty
people. And then the officers came in. They were shouting. They
forced the door and picked up everyone in the room. They had guns.
Only me and my mum's friend Ariam got away. He was dragging
me; I was confused and in shock. One week later I was in London.'

The Human Rights Watch website confirms that the Eritrean government has a track record of religious persecution. Jehovah's
Witnesses, it says, have been especially mistreated.

'When I came to this country I was told it was a holiday,' explains
Liah. Ariam told her everything would be back to normal in a week
or two. 'He said my mum would be released by the time we got
home,' she says, 'but it's been fourteen years now and I haven't seen
her since she was arrested.'

Liah says Ariam took her to Kensington and Notting Hill. He
bought her ice cream. They stayed in a hotel. And at no point did
Ariam explain what was going on, not even when he took her, on the
last day of their supposed holiday, to a social services building. 'He
told me to wait at reception,' says Liah. 'He said there was an Ethi-
opian restaurant across the road and he would be waiting there, but

he must have spoken to the social workers beforehand because they quickly took me on. When I was taken to the children's home, that's when I thought, "I'm not going back to Eritrea." '

Liah spent the remaining part of her childhood in London's care system, moving between foster families and shared accommodation – an experience that took a high toll on her health.

'I was so stressed. I kept getting sick,' she says. At one point a severe bout of shingles landed her in hospital. 'My temperature was so high, I was throwing up, I got really weak. I had a rash on my back and side.' Eventually a blood test revealed the hidden cause of her recurrent infections. Thinking about it today stirs deep emotions. 'I still hate that hospital now.'

The diagnosis Liah was given threw her into a turmoil she has still to resolve.

'Now I know there were some secrets in my family,' she tells me, with a level gaze. 'I always thought it was strange what happened to my father. I had always been told that he had died of a heart attack, but he was very young and there was no history in my family of heart problems. So when I found out I was HIV positive it immediately made me think they had lied to me. They must have known. What made me angry was I was born with HIV and I wasn't treated for so many years. I don't know why they kept it from me. I mean, thank God, when I went to school I could have done something and infected someone without knowing. Thank God I didn't do that.'

From Liah's description it sounds as though she was firmly in denial about the diagnosis as a teenager. She struggled to rationalize what her condition might mean or how she would need to manage it.

'I was so angry,' she says. 'There would be nurses trying to contact me, trying to help me understand the treatment, but I was so ashamed. I hated myself. I was working, I was studying. I really didn't give a chance to anyone to talk to me about the HIV. I would get pissed off if someone mentioned it. That's how I ended up in hospital again.'

Progressive multifocal leukoencephalopathy, or PML, is not a condition I've come across before meeting Liah. With her help and a little research, I come to understand that it's a degenerative disease that takes hold when HIV disrupts the immune system, releasing viruses that are often present but benign in the healthy body.

Similar to multiple sclerosis, PML strips the brain's neurons of the protective myelin sheaths that surround them, causing a breakdown in their ability to carry messages. Unlike MS, which is often pro-tracted over many years, PML kills between 30 and 50 per cent of its victims within three months of diagnosis.

'The doctors didn't find out I had the PML for a long time because they thought I had tuberculosis,' says Liah. 'I kept getting worse. I was afraid to go to sleep because I thought I would die in the night. After two weeks my legs wouldn't work. I got out of bed and just fell over. I was throwing everything up, even a little water. They tried to give me medicine through a tube in my nose but I began choking on it. There was a point where I went without eating for three days.'

After many weeks in hospital, with her condition still worsening, Liah was finally moved to a hospice. 'They literally gave up on me,' she says. 'I was given two weeks to live. Thankfully a trainee doctor who was volunteering there, she went out of her way to help me.'

It makes sense. Imagine being a trainee doctor and encountering someone your own age dying of an unknown infection in a hospice. You would put the time in, surely.

'It's funny because I was treating everyone so horribly. I'm quite surprised she took the trouble over me,' says Liah. 'I was so angry. I can't explain it. I hated everything.'

'You'd been told you were going to die,' I say, 'of course you were angry.'

'Actually I wasn't directly told,' she replies. 'I overheard someone talking about it outside my room. They thought they had closed the door, but I could still hear them.'

How do you respond to this kind of story? What's the normal way to react? I can only muster variations on disbelief, horror, astonish-ment. My jaw drops, I shake my head, I begin running out of adequate body language.

By the time the PML was finally diagnosed, Liah had been in hos-pital for five months.

With the right treatment she recovered quickly but she was left with a number of significant impairments: her memory was less reliable and she now took longer than before to make decisions. Her legs were so weak that she couldn't walk, and her arms and hands had become shaky and weak too. Her control over the muscles in her throat had also been affected, making her speech slurred and slower than before.

It was decided she would live in a care home in north-east London, her place funded by social services.

'From an early stage I wanted to get out of there,' she says. 'I hated it. I was the youngest person there and the only person trying to get better. I had no freedom. I didn't want my life to be like that. I wanted to see what was out there for me.'

It wasn't simply her yearning for a fuller life that was motivating her. 'I was scared of some of the other residents,' she says. 'At one point one of them started coming into my room at night. The first time I managed to talk to him and he went away, but I knew he could get really aggressive. There were only two night staff and they used to ignore the alarm if you pressed it because some residents would use it just to get attention. One time I went down to the sitting room and the staff were asleep on the sofa while the alarm was going off.'

'The council told me to apply for my own housing. It took a long time to do the form and to get their response, but when it came the answer was no. They said I hadn't been living in the borough for long enough. I was told to try another borough nearby and the same thing happened. I was so stressed out. I felt like there was no one to help me. I felt like the council had just left me there for ever. I lived there for six years in the end.'

When she began attending Headway in 2014 we knew that her priorities remained getting away from the care home, finding her own place to live and going back to her degree. But we – and she – also knew that her condition was fragile. Only as long as her drugs remained effective would the PML be kept under control. Any changes that might disrupt her regime, or diminish her weakened immune system, could have fatal consequences.

Eventually a supported-living centre in the neighbouring borough of Enfield was identified, one where Liah would finally have her own flat. The home was run by a private company. The council agreed to support the move. This would be the first time in years that Liah had lived in her own place, her chance at long last to move on from being a patient and take possession of her life again.

Liah moved into her flat in March 2016.

★

Since the first time I met Matthew, his diary has been a familiar object. I watched him carefully writing in it the summer's day in 2006 he came in for his volunteer interview at the old centre. He has written every day since, bullet-pointing events and conclusions and tucking notes and appointment letters into its pages. Each year he begins a new one and the old one is shelved, dog-eared and distended. Without the diary, Matthew would surely forget a great deal more than he already does and his life would be chaos.

But holding the first volume in my hands I feel I'm in possession of an invaluable work of medical history. How many such first-hand accounts could exist, records of the process by which a person recovers from brain surgery only to discover they have acquired amnesia?

It isn't a perfect account, of course. It's only by cross-referencing it with his hospital notes that I can begin to construct an accurate picture of what happened. But that's part of what makes the document important: the inconsistencies are as informative as the moments where the accounts line up. The diary is a fascinating transcription of the thoughts and feelings Matthew experienced and how these interacted with what he was told – and not told – by the doctors managing his care.

The book has a pale blue cover with a patina of scuffing and staining that indicates its age. On the front, written in large black capitals, are the words *MATTHEW'S MEMORY DIARY*.

Underneath this in smaller text are the words *Please use every day*. On the inside cover is a bullet-pointed list titled *DAILY TASKS*:

- *Write down the date each day*
- *Write down what time you got up*
- *Write down what you had for breakfast*
- *Write down what the doctors have said (if applicable)*
- *Write down if you had any visitors, who they were and what their job title is. Also note down if any friends or relatives visited you*

Underneath this is written: *The purpose of this diary is to get you used to using a memory aid and will help us work out the best method for you.*

At the top of the facing page the same person has written the date in large letters, *FRIDAY 1st APRIL 05*. This is three weeks after Matthew was admitted for surgery. Presumably it was only at this point that he was considered well enough to have the diary introduced.

The handwriting is rounded, with little circles dotting the 'i's. It belongs to Molly, the occupational therapist on the ward. I have no idea where she is now. I can find no trace of her online. I wonder if she was aware, as she prepared the diary, that she was establishing a habit that would last for the next ten years and beyond, that would become almost a part of Matthew's personality?

What strikes me first is the document's density. It covers just seven weeks – from 1 April to 21 May – but its ninety-three pages are filled on both sides with careful handwriting. It occurs to me that, at the time of writing, Matthew didn't himself know entirely why he was doing it. He couldn't tell what he needed to record and what he could afford to leave out. In response to this uncertainty he seems to have determined to be as thorough a journalist as he could, to write down everything Molly had told him to and more. Every day, almost every hour of his life as an inpatient, is accounted for. If I wanted to, I could tell you what time he went to bed and got up each day and when he went to the bathroom. I could also tell you nearly everything he ate.

2 April: *Rice, chicken and vegetables. Lucozade, water and hot chocolate.*

3 April: *Some weird mashed potato-like stuff, custard with pie.*

7 April: *Unpeeled baked potato with processed chicken, some sauce (gravy I think), pasta (shell like), custard (normal) with cake.*

I imagine the discipline appealed to him, that it connected with his love of order, with his programmer's delight in detail and sequence. And I'm sure it helped to alleviate boredom. But I suppose also that the diary was reassuring: something to hold on to, a way of reinforcing the regularities in that foreign environment.

It must have been truly frightening to wake after the surgery with no memory of the hours he'd spent in induced coma, or of the days preceding the operation in which he was in a stupor due to the hydrocephalus. As I understand it, the last thing he remembered was admitting himself to the eye hospital at Moorfields on 12 March.

From an early stage he uses the diary as an overt means of orienting himself, to who he is and what has happened:

> *Been in hospital for 3 weeks now. Had brain surgery. Had a cyst on the brain, apparently. Where did I graduate from? UCL, 2004. What did I study at UCL? MACS (Mathematics and Computer Science). Programming languages I have learned: C++, LISP, JAVA, Miranda.*

On the evening of the 4th, after a visit from his sister, Ayo, Matthew writes:

- *Wrote in my diary as Ayo insisted*
- *I (Matthew) need to write every morning, insists Ayo (that would be my sister)*
- *How to get the fuck out of here quickly: Read my diary often, every morning*

The following week of diary entries seems uneventful, giving the impression that Matthew is quite settled in the routine of his recovery. He lists his meals and his visitors. He asks Ayo to tell him his home address and to describe his flat to him. He misses an appointment with Molly and notes that he should always wear a wristwatch to help him know the time and date. He misses another appointment and Molly writes a reminder in his diary herself. Ayo gives him her phone so that he can call her.

He is visited by his old friend Ernest and speaks to his parents on the phone, telling them he is doing 'much better'.

But the hospital notes paint a different and quite alarming picture of the same events. A neuropsychology assessment outlined on 8 April describes Matthew's memory impairment as 'profound' and Molly's notes detail how badly it was affecting both his longer-term recall and his moment-to-moment orientation: 'He was unable to remember his address or recall the date or the purpose of our appointment. He showed severe impairment with recall of three words and three movements demonstrated only minutes earlier and was unable to recall these words or movements even with prompting.'

She notes how disabled he has become in terms of self-care: 'He is able to engage in activities such as washing and dressing but requires prompts to initiate these tasks. With more complex tasks, such as cooking, he requires verbal prompts throughout and constantly needs reminding to refer to the recipe.'

She details how frequently he gets lost, even on the short journey between the ward and the therapy department: 'With prompting, Matthew writes down environmental cues to aid him in route finding but currently he requires verbal prompting to refer to these written cues and is unable to safely find his way back to the ward without verbal instruction.'

And she indicates that Matthew's poor awareness of his problems is undermining his ability to engage in the compensatory strategies she is trying to teach him: 'A memory diary has been set up with daily tasks but Matthew also requires verbal prompting to use this.'

On 13 April the facade he has been maintaining in the diary crumbles. *I got a bit upset this evening*, he writes, *because I thought that I might not gain my memory back.* The downplaying of emotion here is glaring – and betrayed by the reassurance Ayo tries to give him: *My sister was here and told me that everything will be OK because I have come a very long way and I am obviously doing better every day.* Ayo takes him out for a slice of cake and a cup of tea. She encourages him to talk to their parents on the phone. She accompanies him back to the hospital at around 9 p.m. and sits with him for a while at reception before leaving.

It's impossible to know for sure how he was feeling after Ayo left that night, but to me the final note of the day feels terribly sad: *I went to the TV room afterwards and returned to my ward at 00.05 in the morning.*

The following day he is transferred to a different hospital, to a bed on a general ward where he can continue to recover. His evening diary entry suggests that someone has been speaking to him about managing his orientation:

1) *When I wake up tomorrow, relax and get to know my new environment for a few seconds*
2) *Do not react to strange things too quickly*
3) *Read my diary!*

It's a reassuring set of suggestions, but in light of what Matthew was going through, and given the reported scale of his disabilities, it seems a pitiful offering.

On 16 April a good deal happens before breakfast. He wakes at 7.45 a.m. and goes straight to brush his teeth. *Touching my head still makes me flinch*, he writes. *I do hope I get used to it.* He describes worrying about being out of work for too long. *I am restless.*

At 9 a.m. he writes, *Still haven't taken a wash and I think I can now smell myself and I do not smell like a bed of roses.* At 9.15 his morning drugs arrive, after which he goes to the bathroom, complaining of his worsening 'stench'. When he returns, he feels that something strange has happened. More time has elapsed than he expected. He can't account for it.

What follows is a confusing sequence, full of dense and self-referring thoughts: *I spent too long in the bathroom again. I am not sure but I think I might have problems with tracking time without a clock.*

Then immediately, as part of the same paragraph: *Spent years in the bathroom again, I think I have a problem tracking time without a clock, I should mention this to a doctor, it really worries me.*

At the beginning of this repetition I can faintly see that something has been written and erased beneath the text. I can't read the older words but their shadow implies a thought that took a few seconds to write, another few to remove. Just long enough, it seems, for him to forget that he has already written about spending too long in the bathroom.

There is a gap of one line. I infer a moment's pause, perhaps a minute. I imagine him looking up from his diary, taking a breath, looking back. Then he rereads what he has written. He stares at the text with horror. The repetition glares back at him. He is gripped with panic. He writes, *Oh God, no. Read the previous entry again. Your short term memory issue might be worse than feared. Dear God, please show some mercy, I am worried sick.*

As much as anything, I think, it's the failure of attention here that frightens Matthew. It's not merely that he forgets what he's written but that he forgets what he's written *and* fails to perform one of the simple acts that underpins literacy: rereading. For many people perhaps this moment of absent-mindedness would be no big deal, an innocent enough slip. But Matthew was a software engineer. He knew himself to be nothing if not methodical. To the programmer, detail is everything. Absent-mindedness is unconscionable because repeating or dropping a line of code might have untold consequences. The implications of this kind of mistake for Matthew's work – for his identity – are grave.

It seems to me that this episode encapsulates almost everything about Matthew's injury and his own reaction to it. His intelligence appears untouched. When he experiences something he can't account for, he applies his programmer's syntactic instincts: looking for the fault in the code and reverse-engineering an explanation. Time is perceived with reference to changes in the environment. In an enclosed, unchanging environment, like a bathroom, the only measure of time is internal. Therefore, if he is losing time in such an environment, then something must have gone wrong with this internal measure. It's an impressive feat of insight and matches perfectly with Bryan's assessment: the problem is with attention.

Matthew's inattention in writing causes repetition – just as it has in the bathroom – but here the mistake is recorded in black and white. And for all his analytical skills, he has failed to pre-empt the problem. And he sees what it means: *I am worried I might lose my job.*

From here it seems that the themes of the journal, and Matthew's life going forward, are already set. His entries become dominated by vigilance about body odour and dental hygiene, by anxious and repetitious accounts of his cognitive impairment, and by a growing fear about what this means for his future. He studiously records his meals, his missed appointments, his bouts of inattention and problems with

tracking time. He brushes his teeth like his life depended on it, sometimes both before and after meals, and becomes gradually more
fixated on the disorientation that happens at bath times.

On 19 April he gets up at 8.15 a.m. and goes *straight to the bathroom
to brush*. He brushes again after breakfast and tablets. *Also decided to
floss again*. Later: *After lunch I did the right thing and brushed again*.

All the brushing draws notice from the staff but it seems not to
register as anything serious: *Funny*, Matthew writes at one point, *any
time I brush after eating some food, some of the nurses tell me I might injure
my gums*.

At one point he mentions touching his skin to see if it is damp, as a
way of assessing whether he has washed recently. I can't help thinking of the way caged animals sometimes develop strange habits:
circling, self-harming, obsessing over random objects or actions. It's
almost as though the more Matthew concentrates on solving the
problem of his amnesia, the worse his disorientation becomes.

And, behind it all, between the lines, I detect the onset of the
insomnia and fatigue that will be the defining features of the next ten
years.

On 17 April he goes to bed early but is woken by the nurses bringing round his drugs at 10 p.m. By midnight he says he is feeling sleepy
but is overtaken by the banal anxiety that governs his days: *since I
have eaten something I need to brush and rinse again*.

Lying awake, he worries, not unreasonably, about dying. *Let's hope
I wake up . . . after brain surgery God knows what in fucks name could
befall you*.

On 18 April he is given a memory exercise by Kath, the occupational therapist at the new hospital. *I need to think about a number of
steps*, he writes, *write them down and, without the written version, try to
remember the steps in both directions, forwards and backwards*.

Instead of pursuing the exercise in a measured, structured way, he
chooses total immersion. The entry for the 20th starts at 12.50 a.m.
Matthew explains that he's been up all night working on the memory
exercise. *Honestly*, he writes, *I am not doing well*. At 1.30 a.m. he is still
struggling with the same bloody exercise. At 2 a.m. he finally relents and
tries to sleep.

The following day, Kath tells him he shouldn't stress himself out like this. But soon enough, he gets stuck in the bathroom again and begins berating himself: *For all I know it could have been 2 or 3 hours. This is really frustrating.* Ayo visits and tells him he needs to relax. He writes, *She is correct. I really hope I do not disturb her exams.* The nurses join in. One tells him to *relax and work hard* at regaining his memory, whatever that means. Another says he needs to be *fully positive*.

By 3 p.m. he has already brushed his teeth three times in one day.

★

Matthew's condition is typical of surgically induced brain injuries. A very specific, very limited, yet nonetheless disabling 'island' of impairment.

I'm told that incisions that run along the length of neuronal tracts can often be relatively harmless because they don't section the fibres. By contrast, cross-cutting injuries – the ones that break neurons and prevent the passage of signals – can have disproportionate effects, with tiny incisions having grave consequences for cognition.

So, tunnelling through the tissue of Matthew's neocortex, parting the long fibres as they branch outwards from the centre of the brain, Mr Hau was able to reach the upper ventricle without doing too much damage. But as he tried to reach the cyst through the foramen of Monro, he cut or tore across the tiny tract of neural fibres that made up Matthew's fornix, completely sectioning some or all of those delicate strands and causing the long-term impairments that Matthew has lived with since.

It's hard to say whether this kind of injury is better or worse than a more generalized one. In some cases, more profound or diverse impairments can mean the survivor has a less acute awareness of what has been lost. Some of the people at Headway have little or no notion of who they were before their injuries.

I think of Sid assuming he was in prison, or in a psychiatric hospital, laughing gently when I told him why he was at Headway.

Or Nifty, who survived a car accident in her twenties and who, though she retained the ability to form new memories, lost almost all of the episodic memories she'd formed up until that point. She forgot her career as a dental nurse, she forgot her school and college days, she forgot boyfriends and holidays abroad and, save for a few scant sensory echoes, she forgot her entire childhood. The person she was before her injury ceased to exist at the moment of the crash. From her perspective, life began in hospital, on a ventilator, at the age of twenty-six.

When discussing her life now, Nifty says her biggest problem has been dealing with people who knew her before. They typically relate to her as the same person she always was and feel lost or insulted when she tries to tell them that's not how it is, that there's nothing she can do about it, that she doesn't want to talk about who she used to be. 'When my family talk about things that happened before,' she says, 'they can all remember it but there's nothing I can relate to.' Nifty can only look forward.

By contrast, Matthew cannot forget who he was, cannot leave behind the hope of one day returning to that same way of being, of regaining that same mind. In many cases the more preserved your sense of self, the harder it is to let go.

If there is any simple answer to this conundrum, I don't know of it. I remember when I first started at Headway I asked my colleagues what to do when I encountered seeming unawareness on the part of the clients. The answer was always, 'Don't challenge it. There's no point.' If someone's awareness of what has happened to them is low, the difference you're able to make by reminding them is likely to be minimal. For some people the news of what's happened might be distressing; for others it will make no sense or vanish within moments.

Perversely, in more moderate cases of injury, it's precisely the awareness of what's wrong that rehab professionals expend most energy in trying to promote. In Matthew's case, getting him to realize the nature and scale of his memory impairment appears to have been the hospital staff's main preoccupation. Molly's handover report makes a special mention of the challenge:

Matthew's insight is improving but he has many concerns. There is an expectation on him to provide financial support to his younger siblings with regards to education when his parents become older and less able. His sister is at university nearby and visits often but this further concerns Matthew due to the time of year and the exam pressure that may be on her. Previously he was working as a software engineer, and he is keen to return to this role.

I can hear Matthew saying all this, explaining to Molly about all his responsibilities, why it just isn't conceivable for him to be out of work for more than a few weeks. But Molly is clear in her assessment. Matthew can't return to living on his own, much less go back to work. 'He is at great risk,' she writes. 'Awareness of his deficit needs to be further developed and more strategies implemented and reinforced to allow him to live as independently as possible.'

The neuropsychology assessment is even blunter about Matthew's chances of good recovery: 'In the absence of systemic illness, at four weeks since surgery, his deficits are permanent. I have advised the patient that he will not return to work. Unhappy.'

Reading this now, after many years supporting Matthew, trying every conceivable route towards his goal of working again, I am struck by both its simplicity and its accuracy. It seems a weird way to write: using a single word to capture Matthew's response to the bad news. But, at the same time, it says all it needs to. And the last ten years have borne the prediction out with unyielding consistency.

The assessment says Matthew was seen on the day it was written, 8 April. Going back to Matthew's diary I find no mention of the meeting in that day's entry. Matthew notes that he missed an appointment with Molly, that he spoke to his parents on the phone. He had 'custard with cake' and a roast beef sandwich. It seems as though the meeting, along with the unhappiness it caused, has vanished into the mist, the wall of blankness that followed behind Matthew and that follows him still.

★

26 April 2005. Matthew is told by a doctor that he is to be referred for rehabilitation at a centre in Wimbledon. He asks the doctor about the

potential for recovery. The doctor tells him the chances are low. *Honestly*, Matthew writes, *I do not give a fuck. I have to get better somehow or other. Just get the fuck well.*

27 April. *I am low, very low. I have no idea what the hell is happening to me. OK, God, show me some mercy. God, you win. I grant you your majesty. Happy?*

His insomnia and disorientation seem to worsen. He tries napping with the radio on – *blasting away my dreams* – but his night-times are still difficult, with diary entries dotted through the small hours, sometimes describing watching TV until 3 a.m., sometimes simply *awake and confused.*

My soul is crumbled by fear, he writes on 11 May, *and I seek God's mercy by praying but I cry because I am lost, hopelessly so.*

When he is finally discharged on 13 May, the hospital staff are still clear that he's in no position to fend for himself, so, while he waits for a place at the rehab centre, he goes to stay at the friary where he lived on first arriving in London. Two days later he attends church with his friend Ernest. *Got prayed for by one of the pastors*, he writes that evening. *I cried out of anger.* He has returned to where he started. A crushing defeat. He sleeps poorly. He writes again: *Crying bucket loads in my room. It is really because I am scared shitless.*

It's clear that Mr Hau did an extraordinary thing that day in March 2005. He somehow opened Matthew's brain and removed a life-threatening growth from its very centre without killing Matthew in the process. But it seems as though, when Matthew woke from the surgery, the support offered to him began to ebb away. After that intense, life-saving moment of attention, he moved day by day into a zone of ignorance, of invisibility, the effects of the injury on his mental health left largely unchecked.

It makes me wonder: if he'd had the right support, could things have been different? But then I remember: he discharged himself from rehabilitation. It's a well-told story by now because he always offers it as an illustrative instance of his confabulation. The way he describes it, he was offered an inpatient place at the Wolfson Centre – somewhere he might well have received psychological as well as practical support – but turned it down. Instead he went home and went back to work. Over the following days the story turned around in his head and he wrote them an email. 'Why did you discharge me?' he asked them. 'It makes no sense. I can assure you, I'm not well at all.'

Should they have detained him against his will? Should someone close to him have cajoled him into staying? Who should that have been? Ayo? His parents? Ernest? Given his struggle with insight, the depth of his denial about his condition, his solitary habits and his innate stubbornness, it's hard to picture who could have done anything to change the way things played out for Matthew after he finally went home. Perhaps by then the opportunity was already lost.

★

Where did you study? Bryan had asked. *What grade did you get?* What he didn't ask, couldn't have guessed, was everything else that Matthew had gone through to get his degree.

December 1995. Matthew stares out of the train window at the buildings going by. It's eleven years until I will meet him. Matthew has told me something of this time, but his accounts are terse and there's nobody to talk to who knew him then. I'm confabulating out of the box – but what else am I to do?

His eyes flick. There are so many buildings, so close together. Everybody in London lives on top of someone and underneath someone else. He imagines that there was once another kind of city here, like Lagos, with spaces between the houses, and that slowly those spaces were filled in – by people wanting to be close to the centre, perhaps. Or for warmth, maybe. England is very cold. If he closes his eyes he can picture faintly a memory from when he was here before: tracks made in snow by the tyres of a tricycle. He knows he has felt this cold before, back then, when he was a baby, but he doesn't remember it.

The cold he knows is the cold of Harmattan – winter in Nigeria – with hazy skies and sharp morning air. Red dust working into his sandals as he makes his way into the woods. This cold – the London cold – has willpower; it works at you, day after day, coming down from the sky and up from the ground.

The weather has not changed since he arrived two weeks ago. It bit into him as he stepped off the aeroplane. His toes were hurting by the time he arrived at the flat in Forest Gate, in Newham. The lady had opened the door and he had felt the warmth from inside, smelled the damp odour.

'He is in America,' she said once Matthew had sat down. She was speaking about his father's friend, her husband. Matthew's father had not mentioned this; perhaps he didn't know.

The flat was smaller than Matthew would have predicted, even considering how Londoners lived. It had two bedrooms and a small living room. The kitchen was barely a cupboard. The lady was living here with her two daughters. She apologized: Matthew would have to sleep on the sofa. When would her husband come back? In two weeks, maybe a month. What was Matthew's intention while he was in London? she asked.

'To go to college,' Matthew explained. He had thought his father had told them this. The lady smiled and asked if he would be joining them for dinner. Matthew did not know how else he would eat, so he said yes.

The lady's daughters came back from school. They were both teenagers. The four of them ate together and then the daughters went to their bedroom. Matthew waited to use the bathroom. He was exhausted but the sofa was short and it was difficult to sleep. He was woken by the daughters as they got ready for school. After breakfast the lady said she knew someone who might be able to find Matthew a job, would he like her to ask?

He had called his parents from a payphone on the street and explained how crowded the flat was. He didn't feel comfortable taking food from the family. The lady had enough to worry about without trying to accommodate him. She had agreed to let him leave his bag at the flat until he had found somewhere else to live.

He walked to the local police station. The officer behind the counter wrote an address on a piece of paper.

And now he is here, at the heart of the city. Centrepoint is tall and grey. A fine snow falls as he stands looking up at the building.

Inside, the workers point, hold out pieces of paper, push things into his hands. He sits for an hour, waiting for a bed to be allocated. There is a familiar feeling about this place, the hordes of young people moving from one part of the building to another. He gets shown to a dorm and smiles because this too is recognizable: rows of bunk beds. He lies down and suddenly notices that he is very hungry.

Then he understands what has happened. He has come thousands of miles to a completely different country, but somehow he has found himself back at school. He was hungry for six years at school. He did badly in his exams but he was glad when it was over. Whatever happens now, he thinks, nothing can be worse than that.

For something like two weeks he moves between Newham and the centre of town. A couple of times he ends up sleeping rough. He doesn't remember where. He vaguely recalls a house somewhere, perhaps Hackney, with the windows boarded up. He remembers lying on a bare foam mattress in a community hall in Newham.

He takes his two passports out of his bag and holds them next to one another, open at the photograph page. In the old one he is a baby. In the new one he is as he is now: a teenager, almost an adult. At customs they had questioned him: where did he get the new passport? Why was he coming to the UK? Where was he going to live? Why was he travelling alone? He had the sense that they did not entirely trust the newer passport – the one issued in Nigeria. He feels the paper of each between his fingers, looking for differences in quality. Perhaps the Nigerian one is not as good. You can probably tell if you know what you are looking for.

But here is the truth: Matthew is English. That his parents are Nigerian, that he has been educated in Nigeria, these things make no difference to what really matters, what it says here, in ink next to his baby picture. Place of birth: Reading, UK. This little line of ink is what will define his future. His current circumstances are nothing, a minor setback. He will find somewhere to live, then he will go to college. Then he will get a job.

Because he is young he is put at the top of the list for a permanent place to stay. Soon a space comes up at a friary in Plaistow, a tall terraced house with a long garden at the back and a muddle of rooms occupied by a shifting population of young people from Europe, street drinkers from the UK and Christian volunteers who come to visit.

The friar, the man who runs the house, is called Brother Max. He will remember Matthew as a forceful young man, someone who was completely focused on making progress, on building a career, on proving himself. He'll also remember a photograph taken of Matthew at the night shelter in Newham, a photograph that was subsequently lost but which stuck in his memory because it captured something abiding and true about Matthew. There, at the age of seventeen, in the night shelter, far from home, it isn't fear in this young man's eyes but anger.

The Liverpool Street Station branch of Burger King is small. Matthew works in the back, washing tools and equipment, stainless-steel bowls for mayonnaise, for pickles, for vegetables. He is told to keep an eye on stock levels: paper cups, buns, burgers. This is how many we should have at any given time. Once it drops to here, go to the store down the platform and get more.

Matthew stays for eighteen months. Then one Saturday morning he finds he can't get on the bus. He has got up in time, showered, dressed and got to the station, but when the bus arrives he just stands and looks at it. He knows if he gets on he'll be stuck at Burger King for ever. Five days a week, rotating shifts. No study, no prospects.

On his way back to the friary he picks up a copy of the *Evening Standard*.

He signs up with an agency and begins work as a cleaner. The hours are more consistent – evenings and early mornings – so now he can study.

He starts his A levels at a local community college: Maths, Computer Science and Physics. His two favourite teachers are both retired university professors. They are unlike anything Matthew had in Nigeria. They ask him questions, they press him to understand, they present their subjects with rigour and passion and determination, and Matthew feels them pulling at the same qualities inside him, making his mind light up.

You can tell he is beginning to feel more relaxed. Look at him arguing in the corridor with this other student. They are talking about God, one of Matthew's favourite subjects. He is surrounded by Catholics and Muslims, people who believe passionately. He values passion. He is full of it himself but he is also full of rigour. He wants everything, every idea, to be like it is in maths: honed to its simplest, most honest form. If God wrote a book, he thinks, it would not be in Hebrew or Arabic. It would be in maths.

He is a little older than the others and he's ahead in his programming studies, already teaching himself C. He is also relentless in his pursuit of mathematics. He talks with his new friends about the homework they have been set on differential equations. Matthew doesn't just want to know how to make them work, he wants to know why they work the way they do.

Matthew is scrupulously honest. He sets absurdly high standards for himself and refuses to take any easy route. He loves ideas and inspires people around him. He never complains, despite being far from his family and having to work so hard to support himself as well as sending money home. If anything he just works harder. He wants the responsibility. He wants to help his family, *and* pass his exams, *and* learn everything he can. He is testing himself. He hasn't found a limit yet.

You might say these are something like the qualities of a Christian. And yet Matthew refuses God. Sometimes it is testing for his friends, for Brother Max, the way Matthew talks. He can seem so angry about it. Sometimes people ask themselves if it is something to do with his upbringing, or his time at boarding school. Did he lose his faith then, when he was bullied? Or was it when he came to England, when he was made to live on the streets?

But even when he is arguing, Matthew is able to smile. He never falls out with anyone; whether he wins or loses, he always comes back cheerfully, looking for another argument.

Matthew determines that he will go either to UCL or to Imperial College: the top two universities in London for maths and computer science. But he is still working nights and weekends and the lack of rest takes its toll on his studies. He gets two Bs and a C. For UCL he must have at least two As and a B; for Imperial, three As. UCL is the least he can accept. So he goes back to college.

It helps that his job has now changed. The cleaning was better than Burger King but it still required him to concentrate and to move around. Now he's in night security, sitting at desks in the marble-clad lobbies of big city office blocks. He works three nights in a row at the weekend: twelve-hour shifts, Friday, Saturday and Sunday. The Sunday shift ends at 7 a.m., in time for college on the Monday morning. He's tired but in a way it's perfect. He's left alone. He can watch street sweepers under the sodium lamps; he can listen to the BBC World Service. Or he can study for his resits all night and nobody cares.

September 2000. There are just twenty-five people doing the combined Maths and Computer Science degree and Matthew is older than most of them by a couple of years.

He's a little behind schedule – being made homeless, working at Burger King, having to resit his A levels, all of this has slowed things down – but he's here now, at UCL, where he's meant to be.

He sits at the table in the small classroom with the rest of the cohort as the head of department talks to them about what to expect. In some senses, he says, they have chosen the most difficult degree at the university. This is exactly what Matthew wants to hear. He feels at once nervous and excited. He can hardly wait to get started.

The tutor's prediction is not entirely borne out in the computer science part of the degree. Being older, and having thrown so much of his energy into studying programming already, Matthew is perhaps better prepared than some. But the maths is a step away from the familiar, full of baroque terminology and history and with a complex system of notation not found at A level.

The course soon begins to separate the students into identifiable strata. A few drop out completely. Most do their best to keep up, taking a modest position if a module gets away from them, reassuring themselves that they'll do better on the next one.

Matthew sets the bar a little higher. As before, he isn't happy with merely memorizing a technique, or with getting by. Unless he understands what's happening behind the method, unless he can hold the theory in his head and manipulate it for his own ends, he finds it hard to let go. One day, about halfway through the first year, Matthew spots a small group of his peers standing talking outside the lecture room. He approaches them and they pause in their conversation. With no preamble, no enquiry as to the topic of discussion, Matthew says, 'I don't fucking get it. I don't . . . fucking . . . get it.' Nobody is sure how to take the comment: it's both funny and serious.

As exams come around, some of his peers will discover what Matthew 'doesn't get' is in fact a far smaller proportion of the work than many would consider problematic. He's a worrier, a perfectionist. He always does better than he seems to expect.

There are people on the course who are there for career reasons, and there are people who are there for the love of the subject. Matthew is there for both. He is shy; he is a geek. He is also an immigrant. When his peers are out drinking, he is at home or in the library, working.

It's not that he isn't attracted to women. It's not that. But it's not like there are a lot of them on the course. If you want to meet girls you have to socialize outside MACS – everyone accepts that. You have to go to parties. Matthew isn't great at parties. He's tried drinking and doesn't like it. Pubs are too noisy and he can never hear what people are saying because of his deafness on the left. And he's still working two shifts in security at weekends, so that doesn't leave much time once he's done his coursework. Also he loves solitude, the company of his own mind. Anyway, there is still time.

October 2004. Grafton, the company Matthew now works for, is full of smart people: it sets a high standard for its applicants.

Several friends from UCL applied for jobs here, but Matthew is the only one who got in. At his interview, earlier in the year, the founder, Tommy, asked him a question about overcoming a programming challenge but he was too nervous to think straight. Instead he told Tommy about his background – about coming from Nigeria, about living on the street and at the friary, working nights and weekends. Tommy said he could have a job on one condition: that he get at least a 2:1.

He has since learned that Tommy is an immigrant too. He came to the UK at the age of fifteen and started out with nothing. He worked as a waiter in the beginning. This is what Matthew wants, to be like Tommy, to have that kind of success one day; to be able to turn round and say, look what I did.

Grafton run an online platform for trading commodities: electricity, metals, livestock. The program must handle masses of shifting data, delivering up-to-the-minute prices for thousands of different products to thousands of users across the world. The problems in handling so much data are vast and multilayered. They churn in the back of Matthew's mind at all times: while he's in the shower, while he's cycling to work.

The solutions coalesce in his mind like snowflakes forming, as though parts are being filled in by something other than his conscious mind, as though they are revealing themselves rather than being discovered. If he can just see the structure whole, glimpse it for a moment, he will know where to begin.

He explains to a colleague that he is trying to use the Newton–Raphson method to reduce the data set to a more manageable size. It's a mathematician's response to the problem, both novel and ambitious, surprising and slightly intimidating for some of his peers. But this isn't why Matthew is doing it.

He has the sense of being involved in something good, something real, something that he can contribute to. Grafton is run by people like him: people who love thinking. He wants more than anything to do well; to get the chance to do more, to stretch his capabilities. He goes into the office on Saturdays and often works at home in the evenings.

In his spare time he is reading a book called *Light* by M. John Harrison. It's set across two distinct timelines. One of them, in the present day, is about a mathematician whose work will make faster-than-light travel possible in the near future. The other is about a future in which that travel is happening.

The book contains brilliant discussions on the perversity of science. It describes how, when humans finally make it into interstellar space, they are disturbed to find that the alien races they encounter there each have technologies that, though equivalent in function, appear to be based on mutually exclusive treatments of physics.

'Every race they met on their way through the Core had a star drive based on a different theory,' it says. 'All those theories worked, even when they ruled out one another's basic assumptions . . . It was affronting to discover that . . . They wondered why the universe, which seemed so harsh on top, was underneath so pliable. Anything worked. Wherever you looked, you found.'

To Matthew these ideas are resonant of the deepest learning from his degree. The universe can be described perfectly by mathematics even though mathematics is not itself perfect. The greatest propositions, like God, are both true and incomplete.

He now lives in a council flat in Newham. It has a kitchen, a tiny bathroom and one more room that doubles as a bedroom and living room. It suits him fine. Maybe at some point he will have enough money to afford a bigger place, somewhere his younger siblings could stay when they come to study.

On the bookshelf is a row of books he plans to read. He now buys fiction in bulk because reading is the one thing as important to him as work. Some of the books he is reading have been recommended by Rayhana. He met her on his internship at an investment bank during his second year at UCL. These books are mostly not science fiction. Vikram Seth's *A Suitable Boy* is merely the thickest.

He is in love with Rayhana.

But halfway through reading *Light*, Matthew will find that he cannot see the text on the page because his vision has become blurred. By closing one eye he will find that he can just about see the code on his monitor at work, but a thunderclap headache will finally convince him of the need to seek help. The optician will send him to the eye hospital where a doctor, looking through his pupils, will recognize an abnormality in his retina and call an ambulance to take him to A&E.

That same day he'll be placed under anaesthetic and taken into theatre for emergency surgery on the cyst. The surgery, and the experience of recovering from it, will change who he is as a person. He will go back to work but discover that he is no longer able to do his job. A few months later he will be forced into redundancy.

He will still be trying to read *Light* a year later. He will stare at the same page, willing himself to remember what it says, but nothing will sink in. He won't read *A Suitable Boy* or any of the other books on his shelves.

*

Wednesday 1 June 2016. Liah asks if she can talk to her key worker, Bryn. They sit in the meeting room with our occupational therapist, Anya, and Liah explains that a woman called Kate, the manager of her housing in Enfield, visited her yesterday to discuss her HIV. Kate apparently told Liah that she needed more information about her diagnosis in order to assess how much risk she represented to the staff working at the home. She wants to request blood test results from Liah's GP.

There have been some other problems with the home. The emergency alert service – a way for Liah to contact help out of hours if needed – isn't working. The bathroom isn't accessible: the sink is at the wrong height, meaning Liah can't use it from her wheelchair, and the door is hung the wrong way, making it dangerous for Liah if she has a fall. (If you have a mobility impairment and can't lift your own weight, a door that opens inwards can turn a room into a trap.) And the care workers the home have been sending are proving unhelpful: mostly agency employees, poorly trained, unskilled in facilitation, unaware of the effects of brain injury.

So far Liah has coped with these inadequacies, but it seems this latest invasion of privacy has tested her. She is visibly angry and distressed. She asks Bryn and Anya whether she is legally obliged to let Kate contact her GP. She says she feels like she is being distrusted, that Kate is assuming she will take risks or be careless. She says she would never do this, she understands her condition and how to protect other people. She says she feels as though she will never be free of this kind of accusation.

For Bryn and Anya it is hard to watch Liah suffer these feelings of alienation. It is as though she is being re-traumatized, as if old wounds are being opened. She says repeatedly, 'I don't want to tell them any more. Do I have to tell them more?'

With Anya's help, Bryn raises a Safeguarding Alert: a formal notification of concern that can be raised by any member of the public about a vulnerable person and that legally requires a response from the borough responsible for their support. The grounds for the alert are that Kate's behaviour constitutes discriminatory abuse based on Liah's diagnosis of HIV.

In a supporting document, Anya outlines the fact that, since Liah is independent in her use of the bathroom, no staff at the home should come in contact with her bodily fluids. It also observes that any supported-living provider should, as a matter of course, have an infection control policy in place, covering all blood-borne diseases and detailing universal precautions for all staff. (At Headway, for example, everyone is trained to assume the possibility that any of our 150 day-centre clients may have a blood-borne virus and to know how to deal safely with bodily fluids should this ever arise.)

The document describes how distressed Liah has been by Kate's persistent enquiries and requests that the council investigate the concern and get in touch with the home and require no further contact from Kate.

Later the same day, Liah sends an email to Anya describing a telephone conversation with a social worker called Valentyna. Valentyna is temporary; she's what's called a 'duty' social worker, one that deals with issues across cases as they arise rather than being allocated to clients in the long term. Liah's allocated social worker left the borough two months ago.

Valentyna has told Liah that it's time her support hours at home were reduced, as previously agreed. Liah says she explained that she might need to keep her support hours for a while longer because of what was happening at her home. She might also need a social worker allocated, rather than remaining on the duty list.

On 22 June Valentyna confirms that she will be acting as Liah's new social worker and on 6 July she visits Headway to review Liah's care package and discuss the transfer of her case to the borough under whose care she now lives. The two of them sit in the meeting room overlooking the canal with Anya and Bryn.

This is all quite new to Bryn. He joined Headway less than two years ago after graduating with an English degree. To him, Valentyna seems friendly but also somehow absent. She uses a lot of awkward, pseudo-technical jargon that, to Bryn, seems intended to put people off asking further questions. It appears she also hasn't prepared very thoroughly for the meeting. She begins by asking Liah to explain what has happened at the home, to go over the background of her diagnosis and the events that led to the Safeguarding Alert. Liah becomes tearful and says she doesn't want to go over it again. She begins having trouble breathing, so Anya accompanies her out of the room.

Valentyna apologizes. Ultimately the decision is made to reduce Liah's support hours from twenty-five to twelve. As long as the problems at the home are resolved, Liah feels confident she can manage with this.

★

Monday 6 June.

'He's just such an interesting character,' says Rayhana from across the table. 'I think it was just his way of looking at the world.' We are sitting in a small conference room in her office building near London Bridge. I can see why Matthew likes her. She's bright, full of ideas, and has a sunny character that would perfectly balance his more morbid tendencies. She talks incredibly quickly, as though struggling to keep up with the speed of her own thoughts. It makes me feel a little slow, but it's fun to listen to her.

And it's clear that the attraction was always mutual to some degree.

'He always used analogies that made me think in different ways,' she says. 'I remember very early on he told me about something he remembered from when he was a little kid. He said he'd seen this bucket of water and was amazed at this fluid thing that was somehow sitting there and just thought, "This is what God must be." I mean, who thinks like that?'

I ask her to tell me more about what he was like back then when they first met. 'He was very career driven,' she says. 'I think he definitely carried a sense of being the man of the family, of having responsibilities. I remember thinking it was crazy what happened to him, how he came over from Nigeria when he was so young, by himself.'

'Did he ever talk to you about that experience?' I ask.

'He wouldn't talk about emotion very much. You would kind of have to read between the lines.'

'I get the sense that he ruminates a lot these days,' I say.

'He was always a total worrier,' says Rayhana. 'First it was his degree, then he was worried about the internship, then his job. But these things were in his control. I think that's what he hates about the injury – that he can't control it.'

This makes sense. I think about the hospital diary: Matthew's desperation to regain control, the displacement of his agency into obsessive habits.

'A few months before the injury happened we'd been to the Edinburgh Festival together,' explains Rayhana. 'It was really fun being there with him, but afterwards it got weird between us. I'd had a boyfriend the whole time we knew each other and I think maybe things with Matthew were bordering on romantic. I think it was sometime after we got back from Edinburgh that he told me how he felt, maybe early in 2005. And then I'd gone away and we were out of touch. And by the time I came back he was in hospital, so we never finished that conversation.

'It came out of nowhere,' she continues. 'He wasn't sick or anything. I'd seen him maybe a couple of weeks before and he'd been fine. But when I came back I couldn't get hold of him. So I called his work in the morning and they were the ones that told me he was in hospital.

'I remember turning up to see him just after he had the surgery. He was totally disoriented. I remember he was really worried about the fact that his head had just been shaved and he looked funny. But he remembered how he got to hospital. He could explain all of that really clearly, but for some reason he couldn't remember how he knew me. He made some reference to when we knew each other at school. He didn't even ask me, he just assumed I was a school friend.'

As Rayhana describes it, supporting Matthew in the aftermath of the surgery sounds like a lonely and difficult process.

'I remember thinking that if he'd had a core group of five friends that were in touch, maybe that would have helped. I think for a while afterwards he believed it would all go back to normal. I think it was only when he went back to work that the enormity of what had changed hit him. He was very frustrated. But he was still determined. He spent ages trying to code things, just to start learning again. He just struggled with it and got more frustrated. It took him a long time to accept it. Maybe the anger was just a way of hiding quite how intensely upsetting it was for him.'

I notice she has slowed down now, her words coming more gently, with more pauses.

'I think he just closed in,' she says. 'When we first met, when we were, what, twenty, he was kind of optimistic. He felt like he was on track. Things were looking up for him. The injury just came at such a horrible time. He never really got to enjoy that success.'

She's quiet for a moment. 'He always used to talk about a tree. How his life was like a tree and how he knew where it was going and what was going to happen. Then suddenly the tree was gone, and he just felt totally lost and disoriented. I remember having arguments and saying, "Matthew, you have to forget the damn tree. This is your new life."'

What a good friend. So tough. But here again, how could she be sure she was offering the right kind of support?

'I didn't want to give him false hope by being like, "It's OK, I'm sure you're going to get another job." It's hard to find a balance between that and being realistic. I would try to get him to think about what else he could do. Could he work in a bookshop, or could he do other things, rather than coding?'

It seems as though she doesn't really believe these ideas herself. 'Maybe on that point I didn't appreciate the enormity of it all either,' she says. 'Because a lot of the things he used to enjoy he no longer could. The things we used to talk about – movies and books – he couldn't relate to them any more.'

I can see Rayhana grappling with the thought herself as she speaks: the significance of what changed for Matthew. His injury robbed him not only of employment but of the things that made him who he was, that gave his life meaning and formed the shared territory between himself and those he cared about.

As with so many survivors, while Matthew's life has stalled, the lives of his contemporaries have moved on. Rayhana tells me she is about to move to Africa for work. A few years ago she got married. She had a baby last year.

'I suggested he try dating at one point,' she says with a smile, 'and that didn't happen. He'd be like, "I'm too old for that," and I was like, "You're twenty-eight!"'

Rayhana shows me back to the lobby and we chat about her plans for living in Africa. It sounds exciting. I tell her I'm glad to have met her, glad to have had the chance to triangulate some of my thoughts with someone else who knows Matthew. She asks me to stay in touch, to keep her posted about Matthew's well-being if I can find the time.

I remember the reminders Matthew showed me on his mobile phone some months ago:

Do Not Get Married: you are too deeply introverted. You thrive on solitude. You are also very depressed.

Do Not Have Children: Colloid Cysts are hereditary. You could pass it on to your kids.

What's strange about these notes is that Matthew feels they need writing down, as though, if he were not careful, he might just slip up and find himself married with kids. As though, perhaps, he secretly knows that on some level these are things he wants and needs, things he therefore has to guard against.

The way he talks about relationships follows the same pattern. 'I couldn't live with someone,' he will say, out of the blue. 'I just need my solitude.' It's like he's saying these things only because he knows I will challenge him over it.

I've sensed many times that Rayhana might be the one that got away; that to Matthew, for all his determined loneliness, she represents a missed opportunity. But I hadn't realized before how closely linked their misfortune was to the cyst, or the fineness of the timing involved. At the very moment his cyst began to put his life in danger, Matthew was just becoming someone who could trust another person, open up, admit to himself that he was not just capable of love but very much in need of it.

We will never know whether Rayhana might have become a greater part of Matthew's life had the cyst not intervened. What we know, and what Matthew feels acutely, I think, is that the possibility was taken from him along with many other possibilities on which he had, until that moment, predicated his life's meaning and purpose.

When the future is suddenly taken from a person it can be profoundly difficult – or impossible – for them to adjust. It isn't as simple as lost potential. *Potential* is too abstract a word. The future we each harbour within us is as real as the day. It is a powerful attractor, a centre of gravity that gives our lives both shape and meaning.

It is a special and intolerable condition of abeyance that survivors of brain injury find themselves consigned to. In the absence of help or exceptional individual resource, they may remain in this state of inertia, of confusion and mourning and cyclical regret, of failure to adapt, for many years.

For Matthew, as for so many others, the injury represents the domination of fate over his own will. It's a thunderclap of causality that flattens all ambition, all agency, all morality; the imposition of an ordinance outside the human scale of action or thought. The unilateral removal of the future, the denial of the opportunity to witness the more gentle interplay of mind and nature, to fail on your own terms, to choose to give up on your hopes even, at the pace of the animal, within the confines of the diurnal round, across that simple unit of existence we call a lifetime: this is the eruption of forces that belong to the cosmic within the realm of the mundane. It is the intervention of that most terrifying thing: the dispassionate divine. It is a reminder that we exist in the universe as well as in the world.

★

Friday 29 July.

'My preference,' says Matthew, 'is to have the tumour removed.' We are sitting opposite Mr Khoury in his consulting room again. He is dressed exactly the same as last time: dark suit, pale shirt, neat hair. He listens calmly as Matthew goes over old ground. 'I fully understand that from your perspective that's not a smart idea,' Matthew continues, 'that the shunt is preferable. I'm willing to have a go at that, personally, but only if there is bound to be some improvement to my memory and my quality of life.'

With impressive patience, Mr Khoury explains again. 'The purpose of the shunt is preventative because your cyst is growing. Whether you take the cyst out or have a shunt it will not improve your memory or your quality of life.'

'Because my memory is irreparably damaged?' says Matthew.

'I'm afraid so, yes.' Mr Khoury's face, I think, is a picture of controlled anxiety. It can't be often he's confronted with someone so impaired as Matthew, so unable to retain the facts of the situation, yet so determined to put them in such brutal language.

'That's . . . that's a fair analysis,' says Matthew. 'Right.'

I describe what Matthew had said about dying, about just accepting that death would be better than life with a shunt. I recount my reaction: my fear that this would not happen but that instead Matthew would survive repeat surgery with worsened impairments. I watch Matthew's face as I recount this conversation he has no doubt forgotten, but I can't tell what he's thinking. I will never ask him what this feels like to him, to have himself quoted in front of doctors like this, outside his own recollection. There will never be time, never the moment. And he will never ask me how it feels to be the one doing the quoting.

'For me the worst-case scenario isn't death,' I say, 'but a repeat of what happened last time.'

'Right,' says Mr Khoury.

Matthew asks where the shunt would drain to. He asks about where the valve and tubing would be routed under his skin. He asks about problems with peeing. He asks about flying again, about going through MRI scans. Again and again, we go over the conversations he's had with the others at Headway who've had shunts. I tell him they probably aren't giving him reliable information. He talks about the person he met who got better after having a shunt put in, and went back to work. Mr Khoury says that there are many conditions that might be treated with a shunt, that other people may experience improvements, but that, again, in Matthew's case the shunt would be unlikely to affect his symptoms.

'Right,' says Matthew. 'The fatigue will still be there. You see, therein lies the rub because I need some . . . I have to get something out of it. My only objective in life is to get back to work, to be less tired.'

'I think the only thing you'll get from it is the reassurance you'll be safer,' says Mr Khoury.

Matthew asks when the surgery would take place if he agreed to it, and Mr Khoury says there's a waiting list of about a month.

There is a pause. Then Matthew turns to me. 'Do you think I should go for the shunt?'

I hadn't anticipated this. 'I think you should. I *think* you should. I don't *know* that you should. No one can know what the right thing to do is.'

'I've been in this situation talking to people who don't have memory problems,' says Mr Khoury. 'And they too spend a lot of time thinking and worrying about it. It's not an easy decision to make. It's all about chances and possibilities. It's not black and white.'

One last time, Matthew asks if Mr Khoury wouldn't consider removing the cyst. Mr Khoury shakes his head. Matthew is silent.

'Surgery is all about technique,' I offer. 'If you're having surgery you want someone who has practised the technique many times, right?' Mr Khoury nods. 'How often do you perform shunt surgery?'

'It's my speciality,' he says, 'every week.'

'And how many times have you removed a colloid cyst?' I ask.

'Much less often. Colloid cyst is relatively rare.'

'I see,' says Matthew. 'So you would advise against removal.'

'It can be done,' says Mr Khoury with a smile. 'It's an enjoyable surgery. But I don't think it's going to do you good. I think it will make you worse.'

Leaving the building I feel as though we are approaching a conclusion. Mr Khoury seems trustworthy to me. He is calm, judicious, patient. His confession that cyst removal is an 'enjoyable surgery' seems to me an excellent reason to take his word. All along, he's been advising against it. Only now, when it appears that it would help Matthew to grasp the urgency of his position, does he admit that it would be interesting for him to try. Shunt surgery is his bread and butter, but he'd still choose it over attempted removal because attempted removal would be unethical when a safer option is available.

And Matthew finally seems to be accepting the direction of travel. 'I'm taking a bet that I might gain from having the shunt,' he says. A strong position, and entirely in keeping with Matthew's approach to life. He understands what Mr Khoury is saying but he has to keep hope alive. And if this is how he needs to approach the surgery, that's fine with me.

But as we cross the road outside I'm struck by hesitation. It was his question that did it: asking me so directly, *Do you think I should go for the shunt?* I can't shake the feeling that somewhere in the universe, somewhere in time, there is a better option for Matthew, a silent cure by magic or meditation. He is stuck in a world of terrible choices.

We walk to the park and I buy us ice cream from the shining white van there. We sit on the same bench as last time and look out across the green, the trees now in full leaf.

Matthew asks for the third time today if he's shown me the picture of Rayhana and her baby. I tell him yes.

'Always had a bizarre relationship with that girl,' he says. 'Very bizarre.'
'Do you think you still have feelings for each other?' I ask.
'I always did.' His words are both truthful and evasive.

Three days go by. Something sinks in. Something changes. I wonder
if it will stick:

> I think the injury from the
> original surgery is the problem.
>
> My life got saved but I got
> buggered.

★

Wednesday 8 June.
   'When I was a kid growing up, my uncles were quite well respected,
but I wouldn't have said it was them that got me into it, particularly.'
   I'm sitting with Danny outside a restaurant not far from Headway.
The sky is thick with cloud and threatening rain, but there's a clear
Perspex roof over our heads. I'm trying to understand the process by
which he turned from a kid kicking a football into a gangster with a
reputation for extreme violence and connections to international
organized crime. It's something we've talked about before on a number of occasions, but I still don't feel I've got the whole picture.
   Uncle Shane and his brothers have played a shadowy role in
Danny's stories. I know they worked together in their criminal pursuits. I know that Shane was there, standing in the queue outside the
nightclub, the evening Danny was injured.
   But it seems to me that the uncles – and Shane in particular – have
a more pervasive, more complex presence somehow, that they have
more to answer for than perhaps Danny can identify. It's a hunch, but
I want to see where it leads.
   'The only part I'd say they played was taking me to the rave on the
boat when I was sixteen,' he says. 'I saw all the football supporters,
the ICF, getting the respect.'

ICF stands for Inter City Firm, an organized gang of football hooligans based in London's East End whose notoriety peaked in the 1980s when they would ritually travel in large groups to games around the UK on the British Rail 'InterCity' trains of the time. I remember seeing TV footage of the large street fights they would instigate when I was a child, and being glad that there were no major football teams based near my home town.

'Up until then,' Danny continues, 'I was playing football. With the football it's quite lonely, you have to dedicate a lot of time to training and everything. Don't get me wrong, when footballers become popular they get a lot of respect, but it's hard work. These people at the rave, these fellows who thought they were men-about-town, they weren't doing anything. They were just being themselves and showing a bit of aggression.'

'And you felt you could do that?'

'Yeah,' says Danny.

All the same, somehow I'm sure his uncles' influence must have started before this. I ask him what impression they created when he was little.

'You knew they would always be there and look after you,' says Danny.

'They said that to you?'

'Yeah. If I had a problem with someone, another kid or someone, they'd just say, like, "Don't fucking worry about him. If he does it again just smash him in the chin." That kind of thing.' Even via Danny's casual impersonation, his uncles are frightening people. The language and delivery are terribly simple, terribly clear, the intent even more so. 'And just the way that they were around other people,' he continues. 'They were always the popular ones, the loudest. They'd meet in the pub on a Friday, and I'd be there because it was payday and I'd go get my pocket money from my dad. He was a quiet man. My uncles were the ones who stood out, the ones who everyone seemed to want to make a beeline for.'

I picture them standing together at the bar, making noise, full of swagger, unapologetic.

'Did you have any sense of why they were popular?' I ask.

'Because they were good fighters,' Danny says, simply.

'Did you ever see them fight?' I ask.

'Yeah,' Danny says. 'I saw them fight each other when I was about ten. Shane, the oldest one, he bashed up Ian, the younger one.' Danny recounts the memory with a smile on his face: 'It was some family thing, I don't know. Ian was living with my nan, and Shane thought he was taking liberties so he told him to come out on the grass, so they went out on the grass, then they had a –' Danny breaks off to laugh. 'They had a fight!'

'Where were you?'

'I was on the balcony,' says Danny. 'My nan lived in a maisonette, upstairs. They went to the park over the road. My nan and grandad were both Geordies, quite fiery. Nan said, "Oh, I can't fucking watch this." My grandad said, "Oh, fuck it, let them get on with it." '

'You and your grandad stood on the balcony and watched your uncles have a fight?'

'Yeah, "Go on, boys!" ' He laughs again. It's as though it were yesterday. 'Then Grandad told me to get indoors. I don't know what he did after that because he shut the door.'

'And then what?'

'They came back in,' says Danny. 'You could tell Ian wasn't happy. He was scruffed up and he looked unsettled. But Shane, you couldn't really tell he'd been in a fight. He looked calm. He was the more domineering one.'

I ask him if this sort of thing went back more than one generation, his family resolving disagreements through aggression.

'Yeah,' says Danny. 'My grandad – that's where the fighting comes from with my uncles, because he was a hard man when he was younger. They always had someone to look up to who could have a fight.'

'So they probably watched him having fights when they were kids?' I say.

'No doubt,' says Danny. 'They still tell some stories now – how he bashed this one up and that one. He's passed away now, my grandad, but everyone was quite scared of him when he was alive.'

'Do you think your uncles were scared of him?'

'Yeah. I think people of that generation, that's how they solved things, but nowadays they don't tend to fight.' I assume for a moment that he means violence has become less commonplace, but that's not what he's driving at. 'People tend to stab you,' he says, 'd'you know what I mean?'

★

It's Thursday and Henry is drawing at the table by the window. He's working on a picture of a man with enormous technicoloured trousers: zigzag stripes that dazzle the eye. It seems to be based loosely on a picture from a fashion magazine he has found but, like all Henry's drawings, the freshness in the style outweighs any sense of derivation. Like many of the artists that work here each week, he seems unable to make anything that doesn't positively vibrate with originality; every mark is his own.

It's surely partly his neurological circumstances that govern this. But it's the ideas too, the things he chooses to draw. Like psychedelic creatures from *Yellow Submarine*, his subjects bend and wriggle, their limbs branching out, their eyes spiralling.

Before his injury, Henry was a greengrocer. He'd no doubt used marker pens a great deal, but more of the kind you write prices with on bits of card. I have no idea whether he was ever into drawing. I don't know the specifics of his assault – who his assailant was or why they attacked him. Perhaps it was a robbery. We may never find out. It was a long time ago and my attempts to find out have been fruitless so far.

Occasionally you catch a glimpse of the scars above the opening of his collar, or when his shirt rides up as he removes his sweater. I saw them once and asked him, 'What's that, Henry?'

'What?' he said.

'On your chest – the scars?'

'Oh,' Henry said, 'I know. Mad, isn't it? I saw them the other day and I thought, what?'

'How did it happen?'

Henry blinked. He ran his index finger up his middle and said, 'Operation.'

As I understand it, the stab wounds to his chest caused his heart to stop, and the loss of blood to his brain caused infarctions – cell death in the brain tissue. He recovered from the stabbing completely; he's as strong as an ox. His arms are pale and thick, still strongly muscled, with large hands you can easily imagine gathering up sacks of spuds. And he's famous here for his appetite. You can't leave your lunch unattended near him – unless you want it smothered with chilli sauce (he has no sense of taste since the injury) and swallowed in a breath. He's tall and stands straight as a lamp post with his gut before him.

But his movement is slow, every muscle acting at half speed and twanging with a steady spasticity. The impairment affects everything from his walking, which is stiff, to the finest control of his fingers, hence the unique mark-making. And, like so many others, his ability to form new memories has been affected too. In the amnesia stakes he's somewhere in the middle: a lot worse than Matthew, but not as bad as Sid. He knows where he is, who you are, why he's here. But if you ask him what he did this morning the answer will be an informed guess and, startlingly, when he strolls back to the studio after lunch, he's as likely to sit down at someone else's drawing as his own.

Today he is very hunched, his head bent so far down between his meaty shoulders that his chin is almost touching his chest. He tries to turn as I approach, but he can barely manage it, having to move at the waist and roll his eyes to their corners because his neck is so stiff. He's been like this for a week – ever since he was found.

Eleven days ago he went missing from the supported housing where he lives. He was absent for five days and five nights, eventually turning up in a park nearby.

'How's that neck, Henry?' I ask.

'Still . . . a bit stiff,' he replies.

We don't know what occurred in those five days and five nights.

'How did it happen?' I ask.

'Was' – he nods, in as much as he can, indicating something at his feet – 'picking up something heavy. I pulled it.'

It's not a bad explanation. It makes sense of the facts presented.

'It's getting a bit better,' he says.

'That's good.' I look at the drawing. 'I like this,' I say.

'Thank you.' Henry picks up his pen and goes to make a new line of blue in the trousers.

'Henry.'

'Mmm?' He turns again and I squat down to make it easier for him.

'Do you remember anything funny happening recently, anything unusual?'

He looks at me with his very pale blue eyes. They flick momentarily to the side, back to my eyes again. I know that, given cues, Henry will come up with an explanation, a feeling about what has happened – like he just did with the neck. There was a time when a social worker came to assess his activities at Headway. She spoke to him in a room for twenty minutes and emerged very pleased. She was impressed that he was spending so much time cooking in the kitchen, and with the various trips we had taken him on recently. None of it was the case. Henry wasn't remotely interested in cooking and we hadn't been on any trips lately. He had simply told her what he imagined she wanted to hear.

So I've kept the question as open as possible. I want to know only what he remembers.

'No,' he says. 'How'd you mean?'

'Apparently you went on a bit of an outing recently?'

He stares at me, says nothing.

'You were missing from home,' I say. 'Last week. For a few days.'

I'm guessing Henry spent those five nights in the park. In the day he walked around and chatted to people, watched the pigeons. By night he slept on a bench, or against a tree, in a sitting position, his head nodding, which would explain the stiff neck. But we will never know for sure.

He lets out a deep breath through his nose and looks down at the drawing. After a long pause he says something I can't quite catch. I ask him to repeat it.

'Oh, you know,' he says, 'I've got a really bad memory.'

★

Danny's hospital records say that when he was admitted on the night of his assault, his score on the Glasgow Coma Scale was 3 – the worst possible – indicating that he was unresponsive to pain and to the sound of his own name. He had two seizures while under observation. CT scans showed that a mass of blood had collected between the membranes beneath his skull, swelling inwards and pressing his brain down and sideways, out of position.

The surgeons removed a part of his skull over the site of the bleed, cut a window in the membranes beneath and sucked out the blood.

Over the following hours the hospital staff would have watched Danny closely as the anaesthetic was withdrawn, testing his responses at intervals, looking for indications of recovering function. Maybe it was during this period that the dispute occurred between the doctors and Danny's mother – the disagreement over his chances. Maybe he was taking too long to start breathing for himself. Maybe his pupils were not responding to light. Regardless, the decision was made to keep trying, to keep him alive.

Once he'd stabilized, he was transferred to the National Hospital at Queen Square. By this time, the records say, he was lucid enough to point to his mother when asked to, or to the nurse, and to stick out his tongue on command. But he was still on a breathing machine, was doubly incontinent and was being fed by a tube through his abdominal wall. It was also obvious that his mobility had been seriously affected. The notes describe 'spastic quadriparesis': loss of function in all four limbs.

Danny then spent five months in rehabilitation at the Homerton Hospital in Hackney, having daily physiotherapy and speech therapy. By the end of this, the notes say, his speech was mostly intelligible and his paralysis had largely cleared up on the right side. With his right hand he could dress the upper half of his body with a little help and could prepare drinks, although he was still shaky. His left side remained very impaired. He needed the assistance of two people in order to walk. The notes also comment that his ability to form new memories was 'still not good'.

What the notes don't mention is anything to do with his control over his emotions or impulses. The only time they allude to his behaviour at all is when they mention that he was 'concentrating for

45 minutes' in physiotherapy. Perhaps on its own this doesn't mean a great deal, but it makes me wonder. At this early stage in recovery from such a major injury you might expect any problems with self-control to be quite obvious. Some of the younger survivors I've met have talked about how much they hated inpatient rehabilitation, much of the time feeling bored and frustrated, trapped, confused. A number of them tried to escape, some more than once. Given the oppositional stance Danny says he took during his prison terms, you might expect something of this attitude to have surfaced while he was in the highly constraining hospital environment – especially if his impulse control was impaired.

Short of having a neuropsychological assessment, there's no way to say confidently whether Danny's frontal systems were damaged by the injury, whether his trouble with managing stress today is connected to this or to something broader. I had speculated at his house that it might be more to do with a lack of learning in his youth; with the fact that he never developed strong habits of impulse control.

But reflecting on what he said about his upbringing, the culture that surrounded him, the extent to which violence informed even the simplest of day-to-day interactions, I realize I've been wrong. The reason Danny doesn't think his uncles influenced him is because the violence they perpetrated against each other was not just tolerated but expected. It was a way of establishing reputation, of gaining admiration; it was a means of maintaining social order; it was a method of communication, a way of being with other people, of creating meaning, even.

Violence was so intrinsic a part of Danny's background that he can barely identify it as anything distinct from the everyday grammar of normal relations. His problem before injury wasn't impulsivity, it was something much worse: he had learned from infancy that violence was a way of life, a way of getting things done, a way of securing and exacting power. He wasn't impulsive, he was purposeful.

Now he's a different person. The challenges he faced before injury are a world away from the ones he faces now. As a disabled adult and a parent, the demands on him are unusually high. He's experiencing normal stress levels given his circumstances. He's coping better than many might hope to.

★

'If I'm being honest with you, Ben, what happened to me, they should have fucking done something about it.'

Thunder rolls somewhere beyond the blanket of grey above us. Thick beads of condensation quiver on the glasses sitting on the table.

'They try and say, "Oh, his friends should have taken care of that." Yet they're the fuckers who think they're big villains. Why didn't they do it? They're my family.'

Over the last hour, as Danny has spoken steadily about his uncles, his tone has begun to shift from something like admiration to something like anger. When he says they should have 'done something', he's talking about retaliation. His uncles, the big villains, should have gone after the men who beat him up. This gets at the heart of what I'm trying to understand: the culture of violence that led to Danny's injury.

'If I put my cards on the table, I kind of resent them. All this shit I've had to deal with. They say, "Oh, that's all right, Danny will get over it. He's got a kid, he's got a girlfriend. Oh, he's fucking acting all different now." Yeah, why am I acting different? Because you fuckers haven't done nothing for me.'

When we talked about fate at his house back in March, he'd been clear: *Everything happens for a reason*, he'd said. When I asked him who was responsible for what had happened to him, he'd been equally certain: the responsibility lay with him. It was an assertive response and one that felt more in keeping with his essential nature: complaining doesn't suit Danny.

But as he continues, I begin to see a subtle distinction in what he's saying.

'At the end of the day, if it weren't for one of their sons it wouldn't have happened: my cousin who was getting bullied.'

'That was why you got into the fight at the nightclub? Because you were defending your cousin?'

'Yeah. And when I was in prison, it was a family member who did the stabbing and I took the blame for it.'

'The prison term before you got injured?'

'Yeah. I could have got off with that if I'd have given up a name. But I said no. I took all the blame for it. The same thing happened when I went to prison after my injury. I could have given them a name, but I said no.'

'But why?'

'Loyalty,' says Danny. 'They call it grassing. They say, "Don't be a grass." I could have said who did it, but then I'd be a grass. You don't want to be tarnished with that. People have said to me, "But you were in the right." I couldn't give a fuck if I'm in the right, I can't live with being a grass. It's where I'm from.'

Something is finally sinking in, a connection I should have seen before. Every decision Danny made before his injury was driven by a simple code: family, loyalty, respect. And above all, don't be a grass. Danny isn't angry because he got injured. He knows it was his own choices that led to that. What makes him angry is that his family didn't play by the rules.

'I used to be this big person they'd put on a pedestal. People used to get in my earhole about everything, driving me mad. "Can you do this, can you do that?"'

Danny did as he was told. He protected his family. He took the blame when necessary. And then he took the beating. But then what?

'If I said something it was the truth. If I said something was red, it was red, even if it was blue. Now they say, "What the fuck you talking about?" They talk to me like a fucking kid. Like an idiot – because I've had this brain injury. When I was young they used to introduce me to everyone, but now I could be standing there like a gooseberry and none of them mention me. If they know that I know someone, they go, "Oh, you know Danny, don't you?" They'll say, "Yeah, yeah, all right, mate?" Shake my hand. That's it. Over and done with. Because I'm not dodgy, because I'm not going to be of any benefit to them, they don't want to know.'

It's a little frightening to hear him talking like this. After his description of his uncles I worry about what they would do if they heard him now. But Danny seems unconcerned.

'If I'm honest they're probably embarrassed,' he says. 'Yeah, that's what they are. They're embarrassed.'

'They might say different though,' I hazard, 'mightn't they?'

'It doesn't make any difference,' says Danny. 'I've never spoken to anyone like this. Now I know what it is: they're embarrassed. When I see them they all love me to death, they'll give me a kiss. But that's it, they won't talk to me for the rest of the night.'

'Do you think on some level that's because they feel bad about what happened?'

'Yeah, they probably feel a bit guilty. That's why they say, "It should have been his mates that sorted that out," why they get the hump with the people I used to call friends.'

'They don't ask you about it?'

'No. No one talks about it. Even the old mate of mine, whose birthday it was the night I got beat up – he came round my house for a barbecue the other day with his two girls. I went to say something to him about it, but as soon as I mentioned it he went, "Oh, no, no, you don't need to talk about that." So he probably feels guilty that he hasn't done anything. Everyone thinks they can brush it under the carpet.'

Danny pauses, turns his eyes to the road for a moment. 'See, the way I think now I'm a little bit insecure,' he says, his tone softer. 'I get a bit paranoid.

'But I'll tell you this,' he says, turning back to me, his face dark with emotion. 'This is God's honest truth. If I'd known what I know now about how I'd get fucking treated I'd grass them cunts up. That's what I'd do.'

A car drives past on the cobbles and for a moment the air is full of sound and rain. It's as though Danny's whole life is there between us, in the air: all the tension, all the violence, all the promises and blood. Then the moment lifts. A smile breaks over Danny's face. 'No, I wouldn't be a grass, fuck that! Just thinking about it, I couldn't have that wrapped round my name. No way!'

★

I keep thinking about the fight on the lawn when Danny was ten. His uncles are arguing. Shane says, *Come out on the grass.* They calmly go outside. Danny watches from the balcony as they fight. When they're done, they come back in.

It's a testament to the cultural gulf between us, to the differences in upbringing, that when I originally asked him the question about his uncles' influence, Danny clearly didn't know what I meant. Equally the reverse: that it's taken me so long to see beyond my own assumptions about what constitutes a normal childhood.

'When you think about it,' he said, 'I realize I had witnessed violence from an early age.' But somehow, even then, we were not looking at it from the same angle. 'It's violence,' he said, 'whether it's your uncles or not.'

Surely, I think, if it's your uncles, it's *especially* violent? After all, if you'll do that to your brother, what will you do to someone you're not even related to? Someone to whom you owe no loyalty?

Danny had a taste for it. He was a risk-taker with a lack of fear. Presumably his uncles noticed it. It was a congruence of factors, of course. But the messages communicated to Danny in childhood were powerful and consistent.

Watching his uncles attack one another, watching the way his grandparents reacted, seeing the respect his violent relatives received from the community, meeting hooligans with expensive watches, seeing them pull wads of paper money from their pockets.

Violence was normal. Violence was admirable. Violence was something you do to people you love. Violence was safe.

I picture Danny at home with Harry, rolling around and cuddling on the carpet. 'It's hard for me to believe I would be the parent of a gorgeous baby boy,' he says. 'I never thought I could achieve that. He's my world, my boy. My world.'

Harry and Sam have connected Danny to the world in a way that perhaps nothing else could. They have given him reason to cherish life, to keep trying, to carry his burden with grace and be the parent he knows his son deserves.

★

Thursday 23 June.
'How good is that?' says Danny, the pleasure evident on his face.

He's commenting on the fact that Kieran's eyes are open: a new development since he was here last month. It's clear that Kieran would be tall standing up. His long, skinny body fills the hospital bed, all elbows and knees. His limbs look very soft, almost boneless, supported here by a complex array of white pillows and bolsters. Both his hands are splinted and his feet are encased in stiff-looking blue foam supports. I assume these are to limit the impact of spasticity – to prevent the tendons and muscles shortening while he lies here. Becky, his mother, sits next to the bed, both hands stroking his forearm while she updates Danny on progress.

'We think he's sort of looking at things,' she says. One of Kieran's blue eyes – the right one – is partially occluded by a droopy eyelid. The left one is quite clear. He rolls his head softly. His gaze seems unfocused, hard to read.

We're in the neurosurgery department of one of London's largest hospitals, where Danny has been employed for several months as a peer support worker in an early intervention project set up by Headway.

It's the first paid employment he's had since his injury nearly twenty years ago.

The notes say Kieran has been here two and a half months. He has his own room – partly because of the length of stay, I assume, but also because he's only seventeen and his parents need to be with him much of the time.

Becky explains that she's been here seventy-three days straight, alternating ten-hour shifts with her husband, Pete. They don't leave Kieran alone even at night. For a while they were commuting in but that was unsustainable. The hospital has found them a place to stay on-site now, thank goodness.

Kieran is intubated at the base of his throat, via a tracheotomy. There's a feeding tube running to his abdomen. A large depression takes up much of the right side of his head, where the skull bone has been removed. The hair and skin make a shadow here where they sink into the cavity.

'The bone was too smashed up,' says Becky, 'so they threw it away.

They've made a plate to put in instead.' She shows us a photograph on her phone. It's of a replica of the missing bone in blue plastic that the hospital has somehow created.

'Once the plate's in,' she continues, 'once his brain has more space, we might see a bit more improvement, they said. We might,' she repeats, 'we don't know.' She falls silent as she looks at her son. He rolls his head once more a little.

'It'll come gradually,' says Danny.

'They said it was a 1 per cent chance of him surviving when they operated,' she explains. 'So you just don't know what will happen.'

'You're doing amazing,' says Danny.

'Well,' she says, shrugging, 'you've got to.'

She tells us about the day of the accident. Kieran and his younger brother were messing about on a motorcycle somewhere not far from home. She didn't know what they were up to. 'I saw the red helicopter fly over the conservatory,' she says. 'I thought, "Something exciting's happening!" Minutes later his mate was banging on the door: "Come quick! Come quick!" I said, "Is it serious?" and he just burst into tears.'

She explains that the younger brother had his knee smashed. Otherwise he's fine. Kieran came off worse.

Danny asks when Kieran was born. '1998,' Becky says.

'There you go,' says Danny. 'That was the year I had my injury. We were meant to meet.' He smiles at Kieran: 'It's a privilege.'

Becky asks if Danny is on Facebook. He moves around the bed and looks at her phone, helps her find his profile. He shows her some pictures of his son, Harry, tells her about something they did recently for his first birthday, called 'cake smash'. 'It's a gimmick,' he says. 'They give you this massive cake and the babies can just throw themselves at it.'

Becky laughs. It's obvious that she likes Danny, that he's a source of reassurance for her.

There are photos on the wall above the bed, signed pictures of footballers mostly.

'I don't know who they are, to be honest,' says Becky.

'What team do you support?' asks Danny.

'Nobody any more,' she says. 'I don't really care now. I suppose it would be West Ham, still. I like to see them win.'

'Up the Hammers!' cries Danny with a smile.

Danny already looks tired as we walk through the ward – it was a long journey here; something wrong with the trains – but he still smiles as we approach the nurses' station to ask about the next patient.

'Hello darling,' he says to one nurse. I get the sense he knows the staff here from prior visits. The nurse checks the records on her terminal, makes a phone call, talks to a passing colleague.

'Does my head in, this,' says Danny behind a hand.

Next it's Hassan. The notes say he's twenty-one years old and that his accident was 'moped vs bus'. Danny nods and smiles at the nurse sitting outside Hassan's room. She tells us he's just waking up. I can make out his legs beyond the door. Another lanky kid.

'He had some oral morphine,' the nurse says in a hushed tone. And then, as though she feels the need to explain: 'It's for when they get restless.'

There are several family members in the room with Hassan – all women. The nurse introduces us to his mother, Fatima, who steps into the corridor with us to talk.

She tells us Hassan had just got out of prison when he had the accident. 'He was being a good boy,' she says.

The notes say 'decompressive craniotomy': they have removed part of his skull to allow for the brain swell.

'He was asleep for a few days,' says Fatima, 'then slowly he woke up. He didn't speak for four days but now he's speaking.'

As if on cue, through the open door we hear Hassan's voice. He makes a high-pitched keening noise, and I lean around the door to see if he's OK. I can see two of his relatives at his bed.

'He's joking,' says Fatima. 'To trick them.' She smiles. 'He was like this before.'

Inside the room Danny introduces us and asks Hassan how he's doing. A large crescent-shaped scar is visible on the left side of his head as he turns over to look at us.

Danny explains a little about Headway, says that he had a brain injury himself. 'You're doing well,' he says, 'don't give up.'

'I won't give up!' says Hassan with what seems to be mock urgency. 'I won't give up, of course, inshallah. Mum, tell them I won't give up, though, tell them right now!'

When we're outside the room again, Fatima tells us Hassan hasn't walked yet. They are waiting for a helmet before they get him out of bed. They had one yesterday but it didn't fit. And then it clicks into place – what the nurse had said earlier about the oral morphine. He's trying to get up but they don't think he's safe. Maybe he's a little jumpy and impulsive after the injury, I think, liable to sudden moves. His manner is certainly a bit potty, as though he hasn't really grasped what's going on. It could be post-traumatic amnesia: a state of disorientation in which new memories are not being formed, and which can last days or weeks in some cases. Or maybe he's just a cheeky 21-year-old. Maybe all of the above.

Danny chats a little longer to Fatima, detailing the support Headway might offer her. I'm hugely impressed: his manner combines professionalism and warmth. He listens carefully and reflects calmly, clarifying or adding to what people say.

Danny gives Fatima a leaflet and says he'll see her again later.

I say goodbye to Danny and head to the hospital canteen for a late lunch. I find a seat at one of the large windows and look out at the city. Sheets of rain are falling outside and rivulets snake down the glass but, despite the weather, the view makes me glad I'm living in London. It's a strange and beautiful city. And again, as when I was sitting in Queen Square with Matthew, I'm struck here by the privilege of being a citizen under the care of the NHS.

Until quite recently many of London's hospitals were Victorian mazes, some of them very run-down. Over the last few decades a number of the largest and most central have been renovated, some completely rebuilt, costing many billions of pounds. Brick and wood have been replaced with concrete and glass.

London's Air Ambulance – the red helicopter Becky had spoken about, which had picked Kieran up from where he lay after his accident – flies from the helipad on the roof of the Royal London Hospital's enormous new building in Whitechapel. I saw the helicopter once on a practice flight. I was sitting outside a cafe in Clerkenwell when I heard its unique ululating siren overhead, like something broadcast from an alien spacecraft. I watched as it gently cruised by, a few yards above the buildings, and touched down on the church green beyond. Walking round the corner to look at it, I remember thinking it was incredibly clean.

Afterwards I looked up the London's Air Ambulance website: it featured a photograph of a young woman gazing up into a turquoise sky. Her hair flew about her and, above, the helicopter hovered. Next to her in large type were the words *Sometimes you need help from above.* A guardian angel in your hour of need.

London's Air Ambulance is a charity, supported largely by public donation. According to the Charity Commission, its running costs are just over £3 million per year. In 2015 it raised over £6 million to purchase a second helicopter for its fleet, £1 million of which came as a grant from the UK government. I understand that the cost of the air ambulance service is several times that of ordinary ground-based response units, and that there are questions over its cost-effectiveness. But it's what we all want, of course: the knowledge that, should the worst ever happen, help will arrive as quickly as possible. And maybe there is no price tag to a life saved.

I remember reading the transcript of an interview a colleague had conducted with a trauma doctor a couple of years ago as part of Headway's life-stories project. The doctor describes the techniques – both physical and organizational – that have been established in emergency departments to minimize loss of life. He describes how the CT and MRI scanners have been brought into the emergency department for easy access and how the teams have established strict protocols aimed at keeping time-wastage to a minimum and governing what information is communicated, by whom and when. Just as important, he explains, is what information is *not* communicated.

'There was a time when paramedics would come in and say things like, "This guy tried to rape a girl" or "He caused the accident." And even though no hospital staff would ever consciously change their approach, you could see it affected their attitudes. So now, when a new patient arrives, the team lead will call for quiet, then the paramedics will give name, age and a rundown of injuries and treatment so far, and that's it.'

He emphasizes the point of all this: 'Our statistics are excellent. We are saving more lives than ever before.'

The most extraordinary part of the interview, though, is when my colleague asks the doctor about longer-term outcomes. Is he ever asked to consider what happens to patients once they're discharged? For the first time in forty minutes the doctor falls silent. It's as though nobody has ever asked him this question before. The answer when it finally comes is simple: 'No.'

I think about Hassan lying restless in bed. What did Danny say to him? *Don't give up.* Hassan seemed to be in high spirits. *I won't give up, of course!* I wonder if giving up might not be the main worry. One of the traps that befalls young brain injury survivors once they're back in the community is that of criminalization. Once they recover they may be mobile and full of energy, sometimes with modest or negligible physical impairments but with a raft of less visible problems, including damage to the frontal lobes, which are responsible for planning, empathy, consequential thinking – all the things that keep you out of prison.

In Hassan's case the fact that he has a previous conviction makes me worry all the more about his future. Constructing a meaningful life after brain injury is hard enough without friends encouraging you back to old criminal habits.

I imagine Hassan is exactly the sort of person Danny could work with more closely as a mentor a little further down the line, if Hassan would sign up for it.

At least for Hassan there is a prospect of living a life most of us might recognize. He'll be able to walk, I'm sure of it. His talking is good. It seems much of his character has been preserved.

For Kieran the prospects are much murkier. Danny told me he's been referred to a unit for people in low-awareness states but they only take adults. Kieran's eighteenth birthday isn't until the end of the year, so it's not clear where he will go. This is the kind of question that will keep his parents busy in the short-to-medium term. It will help keep their minds off the much larger questions that are surely overshadowing their lives now. How much more recovery can be expected? What will happen to Kieran in the long term? When, if ever, will their son come back to them?

The indicators used to predict outcome after brain injury include length and depth of coma, length of post-traumatic amnesia, and the nature of the injury itself. Based on these, Kieran's chances of returning to the life he had before, of growing into the person he would have been, aren't good. That future is almost certainly gone now, vanished as though it had never been.

Kieran's mother, Becky, didn't take her hand away from his arm the whole time we were in the room. She seemed incredibly strong, incredibly cheerful. I can't help wondering what processes are at play in her mind. How much does she understand of what has happened to her boy? How much can she confront it at this stage? How and when does that kind of awareness develop? How much awareness can be good for a person in her position?

*

I keep thinking about a story I read a long time ago: the tale of Orpheus, the son of Apollo, and his lover Eurydice who is killed on their wedding day by a snake bite. Overcome, Orpheus travels to the underworld to meet its rulers, Hades and Persephone, and beg for Eurydice's return. He sings them a song so beautiful that the dead gather around and weep.

Hades and Persephone give their consent that Eurydice should return to the land of the living on condition that Orpheus lead her into the light himself and that he not look back before they are both safely home. Orpheus sets out on the long ascent, having to trust that Eurydice is indeed following him through the soundless night. He fixes his eyes ahead, forcing himself onwards, fighting the terrible urge to look back. But as he is about to reach the world above he turns. He glimpses Eurydice but she is instantly pulled back into the underworld. As she disappears he reaches out to snatch at her but his hand passes through her wrist as though it were air.

Sitting with a person in coma, we feel that there is a separation at play, that their consciousness is not destroyed but elsewhere, at one remove from their body, from us, from *here*. They have moved away from their own surface – from the sensations that connect them to the world – and gone down, telescoping somehow into a distance that can't be described by normal relations. They are in a place of dream or shadow.

This kind of separation evades our understanding. We imagine that our voices might carry, if the wind is right. But more urgent is the desire to follow, to go in search of the loved one, wherever they have gone. Like Orpheus, we want to go down into the shadows and find the person, reach out, guide them back to the light.

Even Orpheus, protected by the gods, fails at the last moment by looking back to check on his beloved. Who wouldn't? Who could pass this ridiculous trial, this arbitrary test of faith?

Perhaps there is some test Becky can pass. If she stays at Kieran's side long enough: one hundred days? Two hundred? If she touches him unfailingly, if she doesn't break contact? If she says his name a thousand times? If she goes without sleep? There must be something she can do, if her will, her self-sacrifice, is great enough, that will bring her son back. I believe she might succeed where Orpheus failed, if only her test were the same.

★

When I saw Meg next, all the equipment had gone. She was free from tubes and lines and was breathing gently for herself. It seemed she had reached some kind of equilibrium. But I knew now that her recovery had ended, that something terrible had happened, something that couldn't have been avoided and couldn't be reversed.

The clearest picture I have in my mind is of Meg lying very quietly on her back, eyes closed, while a nurse carefully pushed a little pink sponge on the end of a white stick around her mouth. Meg looked very sunken, very heavy, her skin sagging towards the mattress. It was another moment of strange intimacy that made me feel uncomfortable: Meg utterly vulnerable again, transformed from everything that had defined her in life before the stroke. It was hard for me to look at her without feeling ashamed, without feeling that I owed it to her not to see her like this.

Then I saw her move. Her head remaining quite still, she took the little sponge between her teeth and chewed on it momentarily, rolling and squashing it with what appeared to be a muscular satisfaction, the way someone chews chewing gum. Water bled from the sponge and I heard Meg swallow.

'It's just reflex,' said the nurse, noticing my gaze.

Just reflex. I described the movement to Nora, Headway's physiotherapist, and she gave it a name: *bruxism*. It's from the Greek for 'biting'.

At the time I simply accepted what the nurse said, but the image remains with me nonetheless because in that moment Meg became full of intent. The movement was charged with sensation and life. It was almost impossible not to infer from it the inner working of her mind, the urgent presence of her self. Yes, she was childlike in her state of vulnerability. Yes, she was clearly missing some vital parts of her consciousness, those parts of her that would allow her to be aware of our presence, to make meaningful contact with us. But in that moment she was unquestionably alive, present, embodied.

I don't know for sure what day this was. I think it was 18 or 19 May 2010. I know that, in the time since I had first visited, John and my dad had been to see her and that my dad had gone up again without us. On the afternoon of the 17th there was a discussion I wasn't present for but which was relayed to me: a conversation between my dad, my brother and the doctors that closed the door on Meg's prospects, that answered all our questions and fears, that abruptly ended the blank space, the seemingly interminable disjuncture we had all entered just two days before. The consultant's notes record the following:

16.30. Discussion with husband and son. I have explained the findings
of the repeat scans in the context of Meg's ongoing coma. I have told
them that she has gone on to suffer a stroke of nearly the whole right
side of her brain and this represents such a severe event that there is no
realistic hope of meaningful recovery. I have explained that in view of
her illness and prognosis we intend to switch the focus of our treatment
from prolonging life to comfort and dignity. I have explained that she
may die quickly or last a number of days. Her husband has witnessed an
advance directive that states Meg would not wish her life prolonged in
the event of a stroke that would leave her severely disabled.

An advance directive: a document Meg had signed stating her
wishes should the unthinkable happen. I have vague memories of discussions in the house about these things when I was a child. The first
decades of my life coincided with the period in which survival after
severe brain injury was first spiking. I suppose there might have been
some high-profile cases in the media, or discussions of the ethics on
the radio. I suppose also my dad's condition had prompted Meg and
him to discuss what either of them might want in circumstances
where they could no longer be asked.

It was in 1972, six years before my birth, that a pair of doctors
called Bryan Jennett and Fred Plumb decided a term was needed to
describe the growing number of patients who were being kept alive
despite profound brain injuries that prevented them regaining consciousness. These patients were apparently 'awake' in that they
opened their eyes sometimes, but appeared to lack any awareness of
their surroundings. Jennett and Plumb called the condition 'persistent vegetative state'.

In some ways it is a terrible term, but if their hope was to find a
name that would catch the ear, that would strike a resonant chord,
they could hardly have done better. They explained the choice carefully, with reference to the *Oxford English Dictionary*. 'To vegetate,'
they wrote, 'is to "live merely a physical life devoid of intellectual
activity or social intercourse" and vegetative describes "an organic
body capable of growth and development but devoid of sensation and
thought".'

Clinical understanding has grown hugely since then, and persistent vegetative state has become one of many terms used to subdivide what are now known as prolonged disorders of consciousness.

No realistic hope of meaningful recovery. The qualifiers stand out to me now – especially 'meaningful'. These aren't observations, they're normative assertions. And then *comfort and dignity*. As though we could have gained any kind of insight into Meg's subjective experience of those last days.

It's hard to understand the scale of the paradigm shift that prolonged disorders of consciousness (PDOC) have caused – and are still causing. After decades of research and trial and error in clinical settings, the Royal College of Physicians published a set of guidelines in 2013, attempting to summarize current understanding and offer practical advice for professionals dealing with patients in PDOC. The document is both harrowing and humane. It patrols a shadowy frontier between the worlds of medical science, ethics and existential philosophy.

Its first purpose is to help clinicians distinguish between patients who have some remnants of conscious awareness and those whose behaviours are only expressions of unconscious reflex activity – those in vegetative state (VS).

According to the guidelines, a patient in VS may have a preserved sleep–wake cycle, opening their eyes more often during the daytime and closing them more at night. They may breathe for themselves and move around at times. Their behaviours can include chewing and teeth grinding – bruxism – smiling, groaning and shedding tears. Their eyes may even 'turn fleetingly to follow a moving object or loud sound'. But under observation, none of these is shown to be purposeful, anticipatory or communicative in any way. Patients in VS cannot be shown to have awareness of themselves or their environment, and they have no comprehension of language. As an example, the document suggests that 'a smile specifically *in response* to the arrival of a friend or relative would be incompatible with VS, whereas a spontaneous smile would be compatible.'

In a minimally conscious state (MCS), the sleep–wake cycle and respiration are also typically preserved but purposeful behaviours are also in evidence. The patient may follow simple commands, may gesture or give some variety of verbal yes/no responses, and will behave in ways that can be shown to relate specifically to changes in the environment: reaching for objects, responding to language, becoming emotional in the presence of loved ones. These behaviours may be inconsistent but they will be reproducible.

The guidelines describe a number of diagnostic tools, advising on how to use them in parallel, and observe that a patient's status may change, meaning that the detection of 'inconsistent but reproducible' behaviours might require repeat assessments. In the case of MCS it suggests that, depending on the cause, ascribing permanence to the condition should only be considered at an interval of three to five years after injury.

At only two months since his injury, I suppose it would be too soon to make any firm conclusions about Kieran's condition. I remember his eyes were open when we visited and he seemed to move his head towards his mother once or twice. But were these the 'fleeting' reflex movements of a person in VS, or something more?

I remember seeing Meg's hand move once: a rolling, shrugging motion at the wrist. And there was the chewing of the sponge. But when I saw her again they had moved her to another ward and she was utterly still.

Patients in VS and MCS are commonly fed and hydrated through tubes that perforate the abdominal wall. These patients need washing and passive physiotherapy to prevent deterioration of their skin and muscles. They are vulnerable to infection and their surroundings must be carefully controlled. As one colleague put it after visiting the ward in Putney, each patient can seem like a distinct, complex ecology of his or her own.

And all the while, the patient's subjective experience remains difficult – or impossible – to discern. 'Families often ask what it is like to be in VS or MCS,' say the guidelines, 'and whether the patient is in pain. Patients in PVS [persistent vegetative state] are believed to lack any capacity to experience the environment, internal or external, but complete certainty that primal sensations, such as pain, are absent is impossible to know.'

The legal position is clear regarding outcome: 'Once it is known that a patient is in permanent VS, the Court accepts that further treatment is futile. It is not only appropriate but necessary to consider withdrawal of all life-sustaining treatments.'

This is what the doctor meant by switching the focus of treatment 'from prolonging life to comfort and dignity'. There is no provision for assisted dying in the UK. If a patient is to die, they must be allowed to do so under their own steam as a natural, if delayed, consequence of their original injury.

Minimally conscious state is more contentious. MCS is for some patients a transitional state on the way to fuller consciousness and for others a permanent condition, say the guidelines. Patients in MCS are 'likely to experience pain', the authors state, but may give no outward sign. Under these circumstances, life-prolonging care 'may have negative value for patients who experience some minimal awareness but have little to no hope of further recovery'.

After months or years in this situation, what is a family left with?

A degree of consciousness 'does not of itself preclude the Court from endorsing the withdrawal of life-sustaining treatment for any patient who lacks capacity, including those in MCS', the guidelines continue. 'However, as our understanding of disorders of consciousness has grown, so has the ethical complexity of assessing the value of existence.'

The guidelines bring home the fact for clinicians, no less than for families of patients, that these conditions are new and troubling territories. The challenges are not just technical but emotional and ethical. Some clinicians 'readily accept that if the patient's balance of negative experiences outweighs the positive, to prolong their life artificially only extends their period of suffering; CANH [clinically assisted nutrition and hydration] should be withdrawn on the basis of the "First do no harm" principle. Others believe that withdrawing CANH from a patient who has some level of awareness, in the knowledge they will certainly die of dehydration within 2–3 weeks, is against the basic creed of care.'

If the decision to withdraw life-sustaining care is made, the process of dying can be hugely distressing. Dehydration will eventually cause death through multi-organ failure, but 'Because patients with PDOC are often young and relatively fit . . . this may take up to several weeks', and 'Although some patients may die peacefully, others may show a strong physiological reaction.' There may be 'sweating, tachycardia, agitation . . . roving eye movements, groaning, crying, teeth-grinding, chewing'.

'Managing end-of-life care in this difficult situation,' the document concludes, 'often challenges care staff to their limits.'

It took Meg just two days to die after her breathing tube was withdrawn. In my memory it was much longer. I saw her briefly after she died. She looked entirely foreign to me then. Only when I looked at her hand, her wrist, a more rudimentary part which had changed less, could I recognize her at all.

I cannot imagine what the process of dying would have done to us, to my dad, had Meg been younger or somehow more resilient, had it taken weeks rather than hours.

At 8.50 a.m. on 20 May, an unnamed clinician writes in Meg's notes, 'Transferred from ITU to Ward 2 overnight. Now for palliative care only. No neurological observations. Medications as suggested by palliative care team.'

And quite suddenly, at 2.10 p.m. on the same day: 'Certification of death. No respiratory effort for 3 minutes. No audible cardiac or respiratory sounds for 3 minutes. No palpable carotid pulse for 1 minute. Pupils 5mm diameter and unresponsive to light. Rest in peace Mrs Platts-Mills.'

I ask myself whether she had awareness of any kind, whether she suffered, and the answer is no, I don't believe she did. But perhaps no other answer is possible.

I honestly don't know what I felt at the time this was all happening. I think my emotions were confused and somewhat occluded by shock. It was almost impossible to interpret what was happening. I was confronted by sights and sounds I had no way of contextualizing. Both John and I were, I think, also preoccupied by thinking about Dad – and by trying to work out how we could support or reassure him.

It was only many years later, when I finally read the hospital notes for the first time, that I had a sudden and violent emotional reaction. I had, incomprehensibly, decided to take them on holiday to Majorca with me. I read them sporadically in the sun, at cafe tables, interspersed with beautiful walks through the rubble and olive groves of the island's northern coast. I remember swimming out to sea, turning the corner along the coast, leaving the bay behind, and spending hours alone in a state of numbness on a rocky outcrop. The tips of the seaweed stroked my feet and the sun warmed my back as I watched a cormorant calmly paddling and fishing for minutes on end, so close by I could almost touch it. I remember crying my eyes out on a rock in the blazing sunshine that afternoon, sitting a few yards uphill of the bay at Deia.

I cried for Meg's lonely death, for the fact that none of us was there when she had the stroke, for the fact that we missed her last hours of consciousness entirely, that we never had the chance to say goodbye, that had she wanted to say something to us, her only kin, we were not there to hear it. More than anything I cried at the thought of her without family all those hours after Annie left her at the hospital. Long before we got there she had subsided into a silent place. She had become unreachable.

I cannot locate the moment of her passing. Her death was a dance that circled on itself. Looking back, it holds a peculiar shape in my mind, a grey shell, elongated, bicameral, full of shadow.

I can't know what I saw when we visited each time. I will never know how much of her was there. But even someone's body has value, meaning, however far from it their spirit stands. She left no children of her own. She had no siblings. At her funeral I said something about her finding happiness in her last years. I know how long she had waited for it.

A memory from a year before her death: Meg and I stand in Dad's garden together as she burns her old diaries, years' worth of private thoughts from the time she and Dad lived together. She has a smile on her face, sighing again and again, full of relief. 'It's all history,' she says, looking at me. 'None of it matters now.'

As I look back, the act seems prescient to me, as though Meg had somehow known about her coming death, known that she must, while the opportunity was before her, destroy her history, let go. But I understand that's not what happened. Really it was luck or pragmatism or coincidence, because we don't know our fate. Our stories are written in invisible ink, appearing only as we read.

★

Tuesday 23 August. I'm sitting beneath the old cherry tree in my dad's back garden in Somerset, reading journal papers. My conversations with Danny and our visit to the neurosurgery ward have made me think about brain injury and criminalization. Danny was in prison – a young offender institution or YOI – before his injury. He was in adult prison afterwards, once. After that he cut himself off from most of his former friends. He's had no contact with the criminal justice system since.

But this makes Danny unusual. A couple of years ago I read something about how 60 per cent of inmates in YOIs have suffered a brain injury at some point in their lives – a massive increase on the general population, where brain injury is typically found in less than 1 per cent. Correlation doesn't equal cause, as the authors of the research acknowledged, but a correlation this big should at least provoke questions.

An Internet search has brought up a newer paper by the same people. This one is a meta-study, aggregating data from investigations in both YOIs and adult prisons in several different English-speaking countries, published during the preceding thirty years. The authors point out that the papers under review don't report the same approach to assessing brain injury in their subject populations, making it hard to put the data together for an overall estimate of prevalence. But even so, the summary table creates an alarming picture, giving rates of up to 72 per cent, with incidence of brain injury seeming to increase according to the severity of the crime.

The explanation offered in the paper is the same I've seen elsewhere: because of their position in the cranium, wedged neatly into the cul-de-sac above the orbital shelf, the brain's frontal lobes are especially vulnerable in head trauma. They get crammed and squashed and scraped more than the upper cortex, which can slide gently against the smooth dome of the cranial vault. The frontal lobes are the centres for impulse control and consequential thinking: the functions that help you succeed in school and underpin the capacity for adult relationships. Impairments in these areas, the paper explains, are strongly associated with early-onset and 'life-course persistent' offending.

As well as lacking experience, young survivors are often more vulnerable to coercion and peer pressure and less able to learn from mistakes. As the paper points out, they're also typically much worse at playing the official game: worse at being interviewed by police, worse at presenting themselves in court, more likely to be labelled 'non-compliant'.

Whether brain injury is the cause of the original offending behaviour or not, once it's happened it might seal your fate, committing you to a cycle of erratic behaviour and imprisonment. We see relatively few of these people at Headway, of course. They're mostly in prison or on probation. When they have been referred they've often struggled to show up, to manage their time, ending up losing their places or going back to prison.

It's a terrible thought: a prison system full of young men with undiagnosed or unaccounted-for brain injuries, cognitive impairments that prevent them from changing their circumstances even if they want to and a system ill-equipped to help them. And then there's the cost. According to the Home Office website, it costs between £40,000 and £100,000 a year to keep someone in a YOI.

Reading the paper, I discover the story has an even darker side. About halfway down the column marked 'Prevalence of Brain Injury' there's a number that stands out: 100 per cent. Scanning left, I take in the words 'detailed clinical examination' and 'sentenced to death'. I skim the rest of the article and fill in the blanks. The study being referred to was published in 1988. The investigators involved were a psychiatrist and a neurologist who interviewed fourteen men on death row in four different American states, all of whom were convicted of murders committed before the age of eighteen.

An Internet search soon brings up the original publication. The researchers have been very thorough, conducting full neuropsychological and psychiatric assessments and taking detailed case histories. They have talked to members of the men's families, gathering information about upbringing and medical diagnoses in close relatives. The data is presented plainly, in a series of tables covering separate areas of investigation – reported head injuries, signs and symptoms of neurological disorder, family history, etc. – but the stories told are almost unbearably bleak.

Under 'Nature of Injury', the first subject reports being knocked unconscious in a car accident at the age of twelve and being hit on the head by his father repeatedly during childhood. The researchers report he has a 'deep indentation' behind one ear. Under 'Symptoms of Neurological Dysfunction' it says the subject reports frequent severe headaches and lapses in awareness. Objectively, it reports the subject has lost sight in part of his left visual field and shows abnormalities on Electroencephalography (EEG) readings of his brain activity. The second subject was hit by a truck at age four, resulting in a skull fracture and an eleven-month hospitalization, and was hit on the head with a hammer by his stepfather. He reports dizzy spells, falls and confusion. The neurologist 'suspects seizures', but no EEG data was collected to confirm this.

Another table reports psychiatric symptoms in the pair, including hallucinations and paranoia in Subject 1 and insomnia and suicide attempts in Subject 2. Subject 2 was also hospitalized aged fifteen and diagnosed with psychosis. A further table summarizes abuse history reported by the subjects or their family members. Subject 1's parents were both alcoholics, and both beat him. Subject 2 is reported to have been 'sodomized by father and grandfather throughout childhood'. That's the same father who hit him with a hammer.

The remaining subjects have had similarly grisly backgrounds. Subject 3 fell from a tree aged eleven, has multiple scars on his head, a memory impairment and multiple 'psychomotor symptoms'; Subject 4 was shot in the head aged sixteen, has an indentation in his right temple and many scars on his face and has lapses of awareness and migraines; Subject 6 fell from a roof aged ten, had a motorcycle accident aged fifteen, has multiple scars on his head, has a history of grand mal seizures, left-sided weakness and bilateral tremors, visual and auditory hallucinations, and was sodomized by his stepfather 'and his friends'; Subject 7 had a childhood car accident, was punched and hit in the head with a board by his father, has an indentation in his forehead, has overactive tendon reflexes and abnormal EEG readings, and has auditory hallucinations and episodes of mania and depression; Subject 10 has a deviated septum from when he fell out of bed as a child, and has a visual-perceptual dysfunction; Subject 12 was in hospital for six months after being hit by a car, subsequently fell from a roof on to his chin, was beaten by his father and mother, sometimes in the face, and has severe headaches and a memory impairment; Subject 13 fell from a tree aged seven, has a 'prominent bump' on the right side of his forehead and a scar behind his left ear, has a memory impairment and lapses of awareness, left-sided tremors and right-hemisphere dysfunction and was beaten and 'stomped' by his brother, whipped by his mother, kicked in the head by another relative, and sodomized by an older cousin in early childhood. The list goes on.

Statistically speaking, you might say that fourteen is not a large sample group. But according to the paper, it represents about 40 per cent of the population in question: people on death row for crimes committed before they were eighteen years of age.

I go back to the Internet and find another meta-study, summarizing research on death row inmates. It looks at thirteen papers published between 1962 and 2000 from multiple states including New York (before the death penalty was abolished there), North and South Carolina, Florida, Alabama, Mississippi and California. Only six of the papers looked at neurological function. The sample sizes involved are similar to the first paper: between eleven and thirty-nine. These are prisoners of all ages, but the findings are similar. Between 50 and 80 per cent of the subjects showed signs of brain impairment, and between 24 and 100 per cent reported a history of head injury. On average, that's 70 per cent showing neurological dysfunction and 60 per cent reporting head injury.

I find one more paper, from 2004, by the same authors as the 1988 one. This time they've looked at only one prison, in Texas. There are eighteen inmates in the study – again, all convicted of murder before they were eighteen years old. The picture is the same. All but one of them have a history of some kind of head trauma, all of them show signs of frontal-lobe dysfunction, all of them have psychiatric symptoms, and the majority have suffered some kind of physical and/or sexual abuse in childhood.

One subject is described as having bilateral hemiparesis, the same movement disorder as Danny but on both sides, as well as a speech impairment and signs of frontal-lobe dysfunction. It describes his speech as 'unintelligible'. It says he was hit by a car as a child, fell off a horse twice, and was knocked unconscious with a bottle. He has scars on his face and head. It says he was the 'product of a rape', that his father died when he was a baby, that he was 'whipped' by his mother and stepfather and was 'sexually abused by many men'.

I picture this man with motor impairments in both arms and legs, with his scarred face and head, with his unintelligible speech. I picture him in prison surrounded by other damaged, condemned men.

I look up from the paper, a feeling of pressure in my head.

Dad's house sits on the south flank of a long ridge of hills, looking out across the Levels, the expanse of flat agricultural land that, in prehistory, was flooded for most of the year. The waterways that drain the pastures are silver in the sunlight. It's very peaceful here, up away from everything.

But the world beyond is put together wrong, cross-threaded, full of pain.

I stand and walk uphill, towards the small orchard beyond the house where Meg made her fire the year before she died. I can hear the wind in the poplar trees at the top of the adjacent field, a sound I can hear inside me whenever I close my eyes.

I asked my dad once how he found the cottage. He said he was on a walk with a friend. They came across the track by chance and saw a chimney sticking out of the undergrowth. He's lived here now for more than forty years. Sometimes when I think about it, about him coming across this abandoned place and deciding it was right for him, I find it hard to understand, beautiful though it is. Occasionally I am aware of a presence: a loneliness hovering at the borders, in the quiet spaces beneath the hedges.

Some prisoners, the papers said, are in their cells more than twenty hours a day, cells that can measure as little as six feet by nine. Death sentences are notoriously plagued by delay, sometimes protracted for decades by the complexity and hazard of ending a life. In some states, the number of suicides on death row equals or exceeds the number of people executed each year.

Woodpile, brambles, apple trees, circle of ash, sunlight in the grass. Unintelligible speech.

A noise makes me look up, a low, rhythmic call like something mechanical, approaching in the warm sky from the east. Then I see them: two ravens, swollen, gloss, coal-black, long beaks opening and closing, fine worm-like tongues tasting the air. They move across, circling the north edge of the orchard. These are the ones Dad spoke about, the pair that have been visiting regularly this summer, flying up each day around noon from the small wood at the bottom of the hill.

They move across the hillside and disappear into the top of the poplars. I begin to move, trying to keep them in sight, but a sound makes me turn again. One of them has circled back and now, with a noise like a tearing bed sheet, makes a giant loop of black fire in the blue sky between the two big oaks, forty feet from where I stand. It flaps its wings once, nosing upwards, banks to the left and vanishes.

★

Danny has told me he contemplated suicide frequently in the years following his injury. For a long time he was in a wheelchair, and then only able to walk with a stick. He relied heavily on his parents and saw few other people. His worst period came around the third year after leaving hospital. He'd been told by a doctor that his most significant recovery would all happen during the first two years, but somehow this had turned around in his mind and he convinced himself that on the second anniversary of his injury he would wake up fully recovered. When this didn't happen, he fell into despair. Sometime later he got back in touch with his old friends. He wanted his old life back, wanted himself back. What else could he do?

He agreed to hold some cocaine in his flat. He assumed his disability would make him immune from prosecution.

'Imagine me,' he said to me, 'standing up in court, waving my walking stick at the judge. I went, "You're a liberty taker!"'

On arrival in prison his walking was still very poor. For some reason they put him in a cell on the top floor of the prison. He had to walk down four flights of stairs at mealtimes, holding everyone up because he had to carry his tray with his good hand and so couldn't hold on to the banister.

Other prisoners tended to assume he was a sex offender: they applied the same reasoning he had, that a disabled person would have to commit a truly terrible offence in order to be sent to prison.

The staff lacked training. One time he said he was offered an aspirin by a prison nurse because she'd mistaken 'head injury' for 'headache' in his notes.

He'd felt very vulnerable. He has told me that it was only luck that prevented him from being victimized. He'd managed to make some sympathetic friends who kept him out of trouble.

If I hadn't had my head injury I would have been dead or in prison for life. That's what he said back in March. *Some big, serious harm would have come to me.*

But it wasn't the injury per se that had broken him, so much as the specific constraints his impairments imposed.

When I was sitting opposite him at the cafe as the thunder rolled overhead, he showed me how his hemiparesis had worsened. 'It's because of the car accident,' he told me. I hadn't known about this. 'Yeah,' he said, 'it happened last year – it was just a bump but ever since my tone's gone way up.' He lifted the left hand above the table: it was inert. The pale fingers were closed against the palm, the thumb straight alongside them. I watched Danny as he stared at the hand. There was no movement.

Since Harry's birth Danny has had less time for physiotherapy, for the daily routine of exercises that used to keep him loose. It was several hours every day, just to keep what little movement he had in the left side. Not realistic with a newborn in the house.

★

Another memory: a conversation with Danny that happened several years ago, sitting in the therapy room at Headway, grey sky outside, the canal still as glass beneath the tendrils of the weeping willow in the garden. Also a confabulation of the event he described, still more years into the past, a moment I didn't witness but have now as an image in my mind.

'It was at the Dallas Kebab House on Hackney Road,' says Danny, 'do you know it?'

'I'm not sure.'

'I don't know if it's still down there,' he continues. 'They used to do karaoke in the basement, so you could go there after you'd been on a night out. This one night I was down there with this boy I knew from Bethnal Green – one of the boys I knew from when we were kids, when we'd always go out clubbing and fighting. But this is after my injury, this is only a few years ago now. We're down there and there's this guy who's really drunk, falling all over the place. The geezer's getting a bit lairy, getting in people's faces. Then we've ordered a cab and the same geezer's tried to nick it and now this boy I know is having a fight with him. I'm trying to stop it but everyone's holding me back, saying I'll get hurt.'

I can see the greasy pavement, lit by sodium. I can see Danny, pulling away from his friends.

'So now they're going toe-to-toe, smashing the life out of each other, blood off both their faces.' The swinging motion of a head, a pale unshaven jaw, saliva and ruddy fingers.

'The guy who has tried to nick the cab has ended up on the floor, so now I'm thinking there's an end to it. But now my friend has started trying to jump on his head.'

Danny pauses.

'It's terrible this,' he says, 'you'll probably be shocked but when I used to have a fight I used to always try and kick them in the head.' His chest opens, his eyes shining. 'Booting someone in the head was lovely.' I can see the excitement in his body. He lets out a slow breath and the glimmer fades. 'It's terrible. I know what it means to kick someone in the head – now I do. I went, "Fuck this." I went, "Oi! Get off him! What do you think happened to me?" My friend apologized after but that's not the point. He should have known.

'It makes me sick some of what I did when I was a kid,' he says. 'If I'd known then what I know now I'd never have done it. Never in a million years.'

★

I don't know when this happened. In my memory it's a sunny day and Matthew and I are walking up Hoxton Street on our way back to Headway from some meeting or other. We are talking about Danny. The two of them get along well. They seem to regard one another with a mixture of bafflement and admiration. They are so different and yet share so much – fellow travellers. Today Matthew is mulling over the question of family, for the thousandth time.

'I don't know how Danny does it,' he says.

'How he does what?' I ask.

'How he has a family. How he can manage it.'

'I don't know. What do you think?'

'He says he has fatigue like me, but somehow he's managed to get it all in the bag. Wife, baby. And now he's working at Headway.'

'I don't think it's easy for him,' I say. 'I think it can be a struggle.'

'But he's still doing it.'

In my mind the answer is simple enough: Danny just has a greater sense of self-worth. He's simply more able to put aside punishing thoughts about what he can or can't offer, to let go of the life he had and get on with the one he has now. But what use is saying that to Matthew?

'Try this,' I say. 'Just imagine you live your whole life according to your rules, according to your idea of what makes you a good person. You spend all your life from now on doing the best you can and striving to get back to work and be the person you always thought you should be and avoiding being a burden to anyone else.'

'OK,' he says.

'You stay on your own and shoulder your problems and never trouble anyone and you deny yourself the chance to know what might happen if you allowed yourself to get into a relationship. And then finally you die and you get to the gates of heaven or wherever and you meet the angel there and the angel says, "Well done, you worked very hard, you were a good person. But I'm sorry: you had it wrong the whole time. The only point of living, the single purpose of existing on earth, is just to have a good time. The only point of you being born was for you to enjoy yourself as much as possible." '

Matthew is silent for a moment. Then he laughs. 'Yeah,' he says, 'it's possible.'

Soon Danny will have lived as long with his injury as without it. Two people, two lives, two apparent identities: before and after. But the two Dannys are not consecutive, not mutually exclusive, I don't think. Somehow he holds them both in one body. He can be consumed with regret and at the same time relish the memory of his life before, the infinite energy, the self-granted licence to simply live, no matter the cost. In some ways this ability to sit with contradiction, to accept that life doesn't make sense, and seize what it offers, has protected him from what ails Matthew.

It isn't that life with brain injury takes no toll on Danny. He is just as exhausted as Matthew, I think. But his tiredness is more physical, maybe, less rooted in anguish. And at least for Danny his injury is over. It happened once, at a time that's receding into history. At least he can, to some degree, look to the future.

*

In July Liah receives a letter from her housing company explaining that they have decided to close down the service. She has until the end of October to find somewhere else to live.

Anya helps Liah write an email to Valentyna, her social worker. In it, Liah says she would like to remain living in the same area now that she has started to feel familiar with it. She says that ideally she would like to move to a flat of her own with support from a service that understands brain injury – a service like Headway.

Bryn and Liah meet with Valentyna on 10 August. Valentyna says it will be difficult to find Liah a flat of her own and that they may have to find some temporary accommodation in the interim. Valentyna reassures Liah that she won't have to find accommodation herself, that this is the responsibility of the social services.

The following Tuesday, the support worker from Liah's housing company is an hour late. Liah tries to call the manager and the assistant manager but neither is on-site. She calls Headway and speaks to Bryn. She says she is having trouble sleeping because she is worried about what's going to happen with her housing. She says she's worried that the temporary accommodation will be even worse than where she is now. She says she's worried about getting ill again because of the stress. She says she feels like giving up. She says, 'I feel dead.' Bryn does his best to reassure her.

Now that she is living independently, Liah is expected to manage her own finances, including paying her rent, applying for tax reductions as a disabled person and completing an application to move the oversight of her care from her old borough to her current one, where she hopes to stay. Her cognitive impairments and the complexity of many of the council's own processes mean that she can't do these things without support. But as the weeks roll past, the housing company's support workers continue to show up late and on some occasions not at all, leaving Liah without the support she needs to make anything happen.

Meanwhile there has been no word on where Liah is to live when she is made homeless.

In September Liah's social worker, Valentyna, leaves the council and a new social worker called Susie is allocated. She comes to meet Liah and Bryn and Anya at Headway. She seems attentive, like she wants to understand Liah's situation. It's not clear how long Susie has been in her job, but Bryn wonders if perhaps she's quite new. She seems less jaded than Valentyna. She takes a number of forms from her bag and rests them on her lap.

'So,' she says, 'at the moment, how many times a day do you need a carer to come and visit you?'

Liah stiffens. 'For what?'

Susie clears her throat, glances at Bryn. 'Well,' she says, 'to help you with personal care or with taking medication . . .'

Liah looks at Bryn. Her lips are pressed together. She turns back to Susie. 'I've been doing that myself for about four years,' she says.

Liah shakes her head slowly. Her complexion has become flushed.

'Sorry to interrupt,' Anya says, 'but I was assuming that you might have had some handover from Valentyna. Liah has had quite a lot of previous assessments and Valentyna and I have had a lot of additional correspondence over the last few months about her needs.'

'Yes,' says Susie, hesitantly. 'I know it's not ideal, but I was hoping maybe we could just start from the beginning? Just recap. For completeness.'

Liah is staring at Bryn and Anya, her eyes wide. Her breathing has begun to quicken. 'I don't think I want to do this,' she says. 'I think I need to go outside.'

'OK,' says Anya. 'That's OK.'

Bryn goes out into the centre with Liah, closing the door behind them. Susie looks alarmed, a little flustered. Anya is confused too: it's not clear why Susie wants to go over old ground like this.

'Liah is under threat of being made homeless,' says Anya. 'That's what we're here to discuss today.'

Susie's awkwardness seems to be increasing. She clears her throat.

'Valentyna and I have had a lot of correspondence over the last few months about the issues at Liah's home and about Liah's needs,' says Anya. 'You should have more than enough information on file from her notes.'

'I'm afraid there weren't any,' says Susie.

Anya leaves the meeting room and walks across the courtyard to her office. Then she prints out the last five months' worth of correspondence she's had with Susie's predecessor. For good measure she prints out a copy of a previous care assessment conducted by Adult Services that she has on file.

Back in the room, Susie apologizes for the confusion. She explains that, though the notes left by Valentyna were sparse, she could see that she had already made some enquiries about assessing Liah for new housing but that there hasn't been a response yet. Susie says she will chase this but that Liah mustn't worry: she won't be made homeless.

A week later Susie is back, this time with a housing officer called Edrick. Edrick takes a bundle of papers from his bag and addresses Liah.

'With your permission,' he says, 'in order to assess your eligibility, I need to ask you a few questions.' He has a cool manner, very polite. 'First of all, we need to determine your eligibility under the Homeless Persons Act. We need to establish that you are going to be made homeless in law.'

'I don't understand,' says Liah. 'They are closing down. I don't have anywhere else to live.'

'We need to establish your eligibility under the Homeless Persons Act,' repeats Edrick.

Liah looks at Anya. 'What does he mean?'

'I don't know,' says Anya, looking at Edrick. 'I think I'm going to have to ask you to use language we can all understand.'

Edrick smiles. 'I see, of course.' He looks at the form and begins asking Liah questions about the nature of her physical support needs, the nature of her family situation, any support she is currently receiving, all the information that has already been communicated to Susie, to Valentyna and to others during the last few months. It's as though all of these people are required to follow protocols that, though they aim at the same outcome, must somehow remain entirely discrete. As though the Liah that needs housing is a different person from the Liah that needs support workers.

As Anya watches, it's clear that Liah's anxiety is rising, her anger and despair surging to the surface again. She hears Edrick ask, 'And what is your medical diagnosis?' and she knows the assessment can't continue. Liah has fallen silent and it's clear she won't be answering any more questions.

'I'm sorry,' says Anya. 'I think we're going to have to rethink our approach. The council have been supporting Liah since she was thirteen. Her medical diagnosis has been on file since she was injured, and we've had a sequence of assessments and correspondences since Liah moved to supported housing back in March, all of which have confirmed her current support needs. I think it would probably be best if some effort was made to share the information you need internally.'

Edrick looks at Susie, his expression unreadable. When it's clear that he doesn't intend to speak, Susie clears her throat and explains that the Adult Services and Housing departments use different database systems. They don't have access to each other's files and the information can't easily be copied across.

Anya is aware that Susie and Edrick's departments are in the same building. She asks if perhaps Susie could print Liah's care assessment and case history and take it to Edrick. Susie agrees.

Edrick remains impassive, seemingly uninterested, as though such practicalities aren't his concern.

'Please be assured that we are all working towards the same aim,' he says smoothly.

Liah fixes him with a tearful glare. 'I don't feel like you're listening to me,' she says. 'I don't feel like you're treating me like a human being.'

Edrick slowly places both hands on the table and leans forward. 'Young lady, tell me,' he says. 'I'm listening.' There is something about the phrasing that makes Anya angry in a way she struggles to understand in the moment. Liah falls silent, the tears streaking her face.

After the meeting Anya contacts a local firm of solicitors. They agree to act on Liah's behalf if the situation isn't resolved soon.

Liah had been due to return to college this month, but with the uncertainty around her housing and the stress this is causing her, she decides not to.

As the home's closure looms, the exchange of emails and phone calls intensifies. Anya chases Susie; Susie chases Edrick. Edrick's replies are short, infrequent. Susie includes a different housing officer, Kareem, in the exchanges and his answers are more forthcoming but still he flounders. He identifies a studio flat, but the landlord wants £800 per month and the council will pay no more than £674. As the end of October approaches and no solution is found, a senior representative at Liah's housing company called Beverly becomes involved in the case. She agrees to extend Liah's tenancy for a further three weeks.

★

Matthew and I go to see a film called *Arrival*, about a linguist trying to negotiate with mysterious alien visitors whose craft has appeared overnight in a mountain pasture somewhere in Middle America. Each day she and her army escort enter a cavernous atrium inside the ship to pass written messages across the pane of glass that separates the local atmosphere from the white mists in which the aliens are suspended.

After some false starts, the linguist discovers that the aliens' writing is circular, its propositions having no beginning, no end, each being delivered complete in a single gesture. To understand the beginning of a sentence is to know how it will end. As she learns their language, she begins to experience what at first appear to be intrusive flashbacks of her past but which turn out instead to be her future.

After the film we sit in a cafe. Matthew tells me that programmers who work in Lisp say it affects the way they think. He says this relates to the Sapir-Whorf hypothesis. Language structuring mind.

'Memory is time-bound from a human perspective,' he says. 'From a human perspective, you can only perceive events from the past. But if your mind is reconfigured by the alien language then the limitations are changed. You can perceive events from the future because despite the fact that they haven't yet been experienced they are available in time. All events are available. It is just your access to them that is limited.' Later he sends me a text quoting Wittgenstein:

'The limits of my language mean the limits of my world.'

I think of a conversation from before. Matthew and I sitting in the park in the middle of Queen Square, talking about time and causation. Matthew told me how it felt to him:

'It's as though your brain is reading a script,' he said. 'The events in your life are already there. I'm not sure how much of free will exists.'

★

Thursday 3 November. I accompany Matthew to another psychology appointment at Queen Square. It's a woman this time. I can only assume Matthew has been referred on to her by Bryan, the one who did his assessment. These meetings always seem to lack preamble or framing. It's as though there's a whole strand missing, the one where we meet with the person who has an overview of the whole case, the person who's managing it and deciding what happens next and listening to our feedback. The way they talk, it's as though the professionals involved are assuming this is all happening. They act as though it all makes perfect sense.

The meeting covers familiar ground. The psychologist asks Matthew what his priorities are. He tells her the most important thing for him is to get back to work. She asks if he has tried volunteering. She turns to the computer at her desk and spends a few minutes looking on volunteering websites. She prints a handful of vacancies out and hands them to Matthew.

Matthew tells her the biggest barrier is fatigue. She asks him if he's heard of sleep hygiene. More papers are printed off. Don't do anything in bed except sleeping, take time at the end of the day to relax, don't drink too much caffeine . . . She says it's a good idea for Matthew to keep all his work-related activities out of the bedroom. No screens, no TV, etc. Matthew explains that his flat is a studio. There's only one room. His desk is about eight feet from his bed. The psychologist says yes, that is tricky. Matthew asks if she has a plastic sleeve, to keep the papers tidy. They go into his bag. I picture them being added to the inert archive on Matthew's overcrowded desk.

I suggest that perhaps it would be good to talk about Matthew's mental health. Matthew acquiesces. The psychologist says there is a group at the hospital that he could join if he likes. She will make a referral.

Matthew and I walk out and buy coffee at the little shop across the road. Matthew has another appointment later on at the hospital that's been reviewing him since his injury, where the confusion had happened last year about removing the cyst. I knew it was coming up, but I haven't seen my dad in a while and my choices about when to visit him are limited. I know that Ayo will go with Matthew this afternoon, so at least he won't be on his own.

Later, sitting on the coach to Somerset, I text to find out what's emerged from the appointment. His reply makes my stomach churn with renewed anxiety:

They are going to set a date for surgery soon. I am going to get a letter in the post.

The cyst is growing and there could be a sudden growth which could be bad. It is growing sporadically in increments. Waiting and seeing is bad.

Ayo was there and is happy for it to go ahead.

I don't know why, but it hadn't occurred to me that this was on the cards. So far the consultant has been insisting that there's no need to intervene yet. The reversal is both sudden and confusing. Did Matthew see the younger surgeon again, perhaps, the one who had wanted to operate a few months ago?

Who did you see?

He has a Portuguese name, or Spanish. I have forgotten his name.

OK. Do you think it's a good idea? Risk of further damage to memory system . . . Mr Khoury has been pretty clear about that.

It takes half an hour for Matthew to reply. I spend that half an hour kicking myself for having missed the appointment.

> I think they will go through the
> original pathway.
>
> Cyst could kill me. Shunt adds
> complications to my life.
>
> I am kind of screwed either
> way.
>
> This is a time to seek some
> faith and trust in God, I think.

I don't like anything about this.

Two days later he tells me he's received a letter confirming an appointment in a month's time for his pre-operative assessment. I ask if he ever told Ayo about the consultations at Queen Square. He says no. I say I think he should. He doesn't seem to understand why. I ask him, would Ayo be supporting him to have the cyst removed if she had heard everything Mr Khoury had to say about it?

> Oh right. I see. OK, will speak
> to my dad before I speak with
> my sister and mum.
>
> We call the shunt another
> option. But likely impractical
> due to cyst growth. At next
> appointment ask the surgeons.
>
> I think you should start praying
> for me.

*

Monday 7 November. Bryn emails Susie requesting an update. She chases Kareem, who replies saying that 'procuring a studio property remains quite challenging' and that he is 'unable to give a timeline'. He says he would be happy for Liah to 'self-source' a property.

Valentyna's promise, that Liah would not be made responsible for finding her own housing, seems to have been built on sand.

To her credit, Susie does not give up. She emails Edrick and Kareem again, asking if Liah will be eligible for emergency accommodation in the interim and, assuming she is, how soon she should apply. She asks if the application can be submitted in advance or only on the day Liah is made homeless and what the application procedure is. A week goes by and there is no reply. Bryn sends another email but again there is no response.

On 22 November Beverly from the housing company emails Susie to remind her that Liah's housing will be closing for good on the 30th. This is a week away now. No further extension of Liah's tenancy will be possible. She asks if there has been any conclusion about what will happen if a suitable flat is not found by then. She asks if the possibility of staying in a hotel has been discussed with Liah and whether the borough will be willing to pay for this if it turns out to be the only option, and for Liah's belongings to be put into storage.

Susie replies: 'This is currently with our housing team. We are awaiting a decision.'

Two days later, on Thursday 24 November, a homelessness officer called Francesca, to whom the case has been referred, emails everyone now involved. 'Just a little update on Liah's case,' she begins. 'Medical form has been submitted and came back with a full response and decision from medical assessors. I will be forwarding this to Homeless Person's Unit Team Leader who now will be able to make a decision on the actual homeless application. As soon as that's done I will again let you all know.'

Anya emails Susie, copying in everyone else:

I am writing with urgency on behalf of Liah Negassi.

Liah is understandably extremely anxious about what will happen on Wednesday. To avoid further distress I would like to request answers to the following questions:

1. When will Liah be notified about whether suitable temporary accommodation has been found?
2. If a suitable temporary flat is not found, will Liah be offered a wheelchair accessible bed and breakfast arrangement with direct and sole access to a wheelchair accessible bathroom?
3. If so, where is this likely to be; do the council for example have hotels they normally use in these circumstances?
4. On Wednesday morning, what support has been arranged to help Liah move?
5. How will her support needs be met in the new property? Currently her support is provided by her accommodation and this will no longer be available after Wednesday.

I look forward to hearing from you.

Anya has been working with brain injury survivors for over fifteen years — with the NHS, for private companies and now with Headway. In all that time, she thinks, she has rarely felt so angry or frustrated. It's hard to watch the effect all of this is having on Liah, to watch this woman, already so isolated, so vulnerable, being so badly failed by the system that should protect her.

Before Liah moved to her current flat, Anya had been supporting her in going back to college. It wasn't clear how successful this would be or what Liah would ultimately decide about her future, but at least the work was a move forward. Since Liah moved, Anya's support has increasingly become focused on crisis management — on preventing Liah from falling into disaster, on keeping her, in terms of her quality of life, in exactly the same place.

And it's not only her own and Liah's time being used up. Anya looks at the recipient list on Francesca's email again. As many as nine council employees are now embroiled in Liah's case. At least four have interchangeable-sounding jobs involving housing, but not one of them seems able to make anything happen, to provide definitive answers or make concrete decisions, each reduced to covering his or her own back while hoping the problem will go away. And in confronting this failing system, in being the only people with a sustained knowledge of Liah's situation, Anya and Bryn have slowly borne a growing weight of responsibility.

Anya is exhausted by it. She has lost sleep worrying about Liah. It's an unsustainable situation but, until some resolution is found, she has no intention of giving in.

Bryn is now twenty-five, the same age I was when I started working for Headway. It's been a steep learning curve across the two years since he started, but he has shown himself to have many useful qualities. He's an excellent listener, a deep thinker.

He was glad when Susie took over from Valentyna. She is young too, maybe a year or so older than him. He likes her. But as the weeks have drawn by and the situation has worsened, Bryn has developed the sense that Susie is increasingly stressed by many aspects of what is happening: by the worry that she is making mistakes, by the fear that she is representing a bad or dysfunctional system, by the likely consequences for her career if complaints are made.

Along with this growing sense of burden, he has noticed a change in Susie's language. Where before in emails she would refer to Liah by her first name, she has recently started to use only her last. 'Ms Negassi' she calls her now. Her manner in meetings is also much stiffer, retaining an air of professionalism in defiance, or denial, of the highly personal consequences for Liah of what's happening. She has moved away from making promises and towards the management of expectations. She has implied more than once now that through its interference Headway – and by extension Bryn – is standing in the way of Liah's progress towards independence, as though Liah had chosen to live without support and Headway were trying to stop her. She talks about 'choice' and 'empowerment', but it seems as though these words have become no more than euphemisms for the withdrawal of state support.

Bryn has also seen the effect Liah's anger has had on Susie. Doubtless not all of it has been justified. Susie is only the latest face of a system that has disempowered Liah by turns. It isn't her fault, but Liah doesn't hold back; at times her fury flashes in her eyes.

As he sits opposite Susie now in the meeting room he feels sorry for her. She is visibly upset but working hard to suppress her feelings. She looks, he thinks, vulnerable.

He has recently been pressing Susie for greater detail about her contingency planning, asking steadily more forcefully about what will happen to Liah if a satisfactory property can't be found.

He and Susie are moving down a corridor whose walls are closing in. Soon things might be said that can't be taken back.

'So what happens,' he says to Susie, 'when this wheelchair-accessible flat doesn't appear?'

'Then,' says Susie, 'Liah declares herself homeless on the day her home closes and temporary accommodation is found.'

'But,' says Liah, 'where will that be? Will that be in the same area?'

'I'm afraid I can't make any guarantees,' says Susie.

'So when will you know?' asks Bryn. 'The day before Liah is made homeless? On the day itself?'

Susie says nothing.

'It's hard for me to accept that there's really no way of forestalling some of the stress and uncertainty for Liah,' says Bryn.

'I'm limited in the help I can offer,' says Susie, 'because Liah is refusing to do her part.'

'What do you mean?'

'Well, if she won't allow anyone to assess her then it's very difficult for me to make arguments for her needs.'

'I haven't refused anything,' says Liah. 'You have all the information about me. I've been assessed a hundred times. My disability isn't going to go away.'

'Look,' says Susie after a pause, 'we can't give any clear assurances about where the temporary accommodation would be. There's housing stock outside London which is sometimes used for these purposes.'

'Outside London?' Liah repeats. She looks to Bryn, baffled, but Bryn has been wrong-footed too. Until this moment the discussion has been merely disempowering, frustrating, alienating, like so many preceding it. But with these words Susie has shifted it suddenly into a zone of unreason, something dreamlike and terrible, dislocated from any previously known reality.

'Where outside?' says Liah.

'I'm aware that there is some housing stock in Birmingham,' says Susie.

Bryn feels cornered. He knows how profoundly this news will affect Liah – knows that she is, at this moment, on the brink of breakdown. But how can he protect her from this news without promising her something he simply can't deliver. The desperate thought arises momentarily of inviting Liah to come and live with him, in the house he shares with friends. But then he remembers: the bathroom is upstairs.

Instead, turning to Liah, he flounders. 'We won't let that happen.'

He turns back to Susie and searches her face. Surely she cannot be unaware of the implications of what she is saying. She knows how vulnerable Liah is. She knows that moving her away from London – away from her medical team, away from the support of her friends, of Headway – is an insane idea. But as he stares he sees in Susie's face only a mirror of his own confusion.

The solicitors explain over the phone that, though local authorities technically have a right to house people out of borough, the law provides for this action to be challenged if it represents a threat to the well-being of the client. There's a strong case in this instance that the action would be unlawful.

Anya says she will book a hotel and a storage unit for Liah's possessions. She says not to tell anyone from social services that this is happening. It's a back-up plan. There's no way Liah will go to Birmingham.

Liah doesn't sleep much that weekend. She lies awake, remembering being in the hospice, being close to death, not knowing if she would be able to eat the next day, or if she would wake up. She thinks about the young doctor that helped her, that young girl, the same age, almost, as herself. And then, when she began to recover . . . that was when the social services became involved again. It was as though her survival was the source only of problems for them, as though she were nothing but an inconvenience. All they could talk about was the fact that she was eighteen now, that she was an adult, that she could look after herself. All they wanted was to let her go. Because she meant nothing to them. She was not a human being, she was an object.

She thinks about her childhood. She tries to remember her mother's face but nothing comes. She had a photograph of her once but it went missing, along with many of her other possessions, after she went into hospital.

It occurs to Liah, not for the first time, that perhaps something strange happened in hospital, something similar to death but less certain. A change, then, into another version of herself, or a transportation into another person's life.

She thinks, with terrible clarity, that it would be better to have died. Better to be dead than this.

She has been struggling with her medication again. The tablets have become hard to swallow. Her throat tightens around them.

She says her name quietly in the dark. 'Liah.'

Birmingham. She can't shake the feeling that the idea has been put forward as a way of pressuring her into accepting some other option the council have in mind. Probably, she thinks, they will try to put her back in a care home.

The day before Liah is due to be made homeless there has been no word on where she will live, when she will be told, or what provision will be made for her support.

The solicitors send a legal notice to Susie and Edrick requiring confirmation that accommodation will be provided within Headway East London's catchment area and that this be sent in writing by 5 p.m. the same day. The notice says, 'The cost to the authority of sourcing this accommodation is, with respect, minuscule compared to the probable harm the applicant will suffer if she is moved outside the area of her support. It is not speculative to say that the move could cause, or hasten, the applicant's death.'

The next day Bryn sits with Liah in her flat, surrounded by boxes of her possessions. In the end, the tenancy for several of the residents was extended and many of them are leaving today. The company has arranged a removals van and each resident has been given a time slot for their possessions to be taken to their new homes.

Bryn and Liah need to be ready for their slot at 2 p.m., but they don't know where they will be going because there has still been no word from the council. At the moment they are assuming she will go to the hotel booked by Anya, so Bryn has called the manager there to make some last-minute checks. He's also spoken to a storage company based locally. He's trying to work out how all of this will fit into the day while at the same time trying to keep Liah's spirits up. He and Liah get on well. He is trying to put an adventurous spin on it.

Back at Headway, Anya has been on the phone to the solicitors. They have agreed that if the council haven't contacted Liah in writing by 12.30 p.m., they will issue court proceedings.

At 12.15, Edrick calls Headway and asks Anya where Liah is. Anya tells him she is at her flat, waiting to hear from him.

'We've found her a place,' says Edrick. 'She needs to come to the council building before 5 p.m. to sign for the tenancy.'

The traffic is slow and by the time Bryn and Liah arrive it's after 4 p.m. They sit in the reception area for what feels like an age. Bryn tries calling Edrick but there's no reply. It seems they must wait.

Eventually Liah suggests they go and get some air. It's cold outside, only a few degrees above freezing, but this is where Edrick finds them, standing in the dark cement forecourt of the anonymous glass council building.

'How are you today, young lady?' he asks Liah.

Liah ignores the question. She has been working hard on finding ways to assert herself, to take control of these conversations. Her sense of injustice and her desire to communicate her hurt are almost overwhelming. She leaves a silence and then, when she is sure he is listening, says, 'I want you to understand how hard this has been for me.'

Edrick smiles gently. 'Well,' he says, 'at least you're not sleeping on the streets.'

The moment the words are uttered, Bryn has the intense desire to destroy the exchange, to wind time back, to have acted somehow in anticipation of this dreadful conclusion. Another moment he could not possibly have anticipated. Another, seemingly dispassionate, assertion of Liah's frailty and his own as her advocate.

Edrick shows them to a desk at which another unknown council employee is waiting with the tenancy forms and the keys to the new flat. Another stranger who seems to know nothing about Liah. His job is simply to dispense keys.

They take another cab to the new flat and are met by a man whose name they both immediately forget. He doesn't tell them what his role is and they are too tired to ask. He merely shows them in.

The flat is on the ground floor so Liah can get into it, but from there on it's all bad news. The bathroom is so narrow that she won't be able to turn around. The toilet is low to the ground and there are no rails, meaning she will struggle to transfer without help. There is a bath but no shower: again she won't be able to transfer alone. All the doors are fitted with self-closing mechanisms that make them incredibly heavy. With her weakened arms and torso, Liah discovers she isn't strong enough to open them by herself. The interior ones can be wedged, but once the front door closes she will be trapped.

'I can't believe it,' says Liah. 'After all we've gone through.'

Bryn looks at the man who has shown them into the flat. Who is he? Is he the janitor? He's not responsible.

Bryn thinks of calling Edrick but the council offices will be closed by now. He takes out his phone, intending to call Anya, but discovers his phone has no reception. He asks Liah about hers. She looks at her phone, shakes her head. They are in some kind of dead spot. This is another blow. If Liah gets into any kind of trouble, she won't be able to call for help.

Bryn feels a wave of fear and loneliness come over him then – and something else that takes a moment to identify: vertigo. It's as though he were watching Liah suspended in space from a thread. He has the urge to somehow stand beneath her, arms wide, ready to catch. He can't leave her here, but he knows he is out of his depth. He looks at Liah.

'It's OK,' she says. 'Let's go back and get my things. Let's get it over with.'

But instead of the darkened building they were expecting, when they arrive at Liah's old home they discover there are lights on. Inside, a staff member explains that one of the other residents has refused to leave. He took all his clothes off and refused to put them back on until they agreed to let him stay.

'Maybe that's what we should have done,' says Liah.

The staff member says Liah can stay tonight too if she wants. Bryn feels a wave of relief and gratitude towards the woman.

Later, at home, Bryn thinks about what Edrick said at the council offices. *At least you're not sleeping on the streets.* As though Liah might feasibly sleep on the streets and still live. To think of it is painful. For Edrick to frame it in words, to share it with Liah and smile, to introduce the image of this fate only to highlight his own beneficence in stooping to prevent it – this, thinks Bryn, is a kind of violence.

Anya visits the next day to help Liah move. At the new flat, with some experimentation, they discover a way that Liah can open the doors by herself. It's still a struggle, and creates a risk that she might fall or get hurt. Back at Headway Anya emails Susie with a list of equipment that will help Liah and asks her to contact the landlord about adjusting the door-closing mechanisms.

A number of emails later, Anya manages to reach the landlord but he refuses to take responsibility. If there is a fire, he says, and the doors have been tampered with he might be held accountable for Liah's death or injury. The fact that, as they currently are, the doors represent the risk of Liah being trapped in the burning flat doesn't seem to figure in his reasoning.

Given the landlord's position, the council tell Liah that they will assess her ability to open the doors and that if she can't safely open them by herself they will move her once again, this time to a hostel.

Anya meets the landlord at the flat. He hands her a screwdriver and watches her adjust the mechanisms.

A few days later, Anya receives an email from the head of Adult Services at the council:

Dear Anya – many thanks for all your involvement in LN's case; your historic knowledge has been very helpful. As you are aware, LN has an allocated social worker as well as a Senior Practitioner OT. You'll also be aware that both of these practitioners are in close liaison with our Housing colleagues.

I've noticed that you've also been liaising with Housing. In order to support Liah we need to ensure there is a clear communication process. If you wish to make any points or provide support please liaise directly with Liah's social worker and OT. I have also related this to Housing.

We are all working towards the same outcome which is independence for Liah. Housing options are extremely limited so identifying fully accessible accommodation is a challenge. We need to ensure that while Liah is in her temporary accommodation we mitigate the risks within the context of feasibility.

In order to move things on I have instructed Susie to visit Liah at home as a matter of urgency to complete her assessment in order to commission suitable services.

It would be helpful to gather information from you that would contribute to this assessment. However, it's not appropriate for Headway to represent Liah as her advocate as you are a provider that we commission. If Liah required an advocacy service we would commission this service for her.

Should you require any clarification please do not hesitate to contact me.

It's unclear how long Liah will be expected to stay in her 'temporary' accommodation, how long the risks presented by this accommodation will need to be mitigated 'within the context of feasibility', or when, if ever, something both accessible and safe will be found for her. It's unclear how the council would define the need for advocacy, or at what point Liah might be deemed deserving of it, or what agency might be commissioned to provide it for her if not Headway. It's not clear how the council, in being so neglectful of Liah's best interests, might find another agency to act on her behalf that wouldn't then be forced, just as Headway has been forced, into the role of antagonist.

Two weeks after the email the council attempts to withdraw

funding for Liah's support work hours, leaving her without help at home. Anya engages the solicitors again to force the reversal of this decision.

'Anything is better than staying at the care home,' says Liah. 'Just being out of there I've got more opportunities.'

We are sitting in the meeting room at Headway. She's clear that she made the right choice, even though the process of trying to find a new home has been – still is – traumatizing.

'What do you think would have happened,' I ask, 'if you hadn't fought to get out of there? Would you still be there now?'

'No, I'd probably be dead.' Her implied meaning is clear. 'I'm not that kind of person,' she says, 'but it was just too much. I didn't want my life to be like that.'

I ask her if she feels like she has begun to process any of what's happened to her, or come to terms with it.

'Some things I think about and it's hard to say how I managed to get through them,' she says. 'When I was diagnosed with HIV it took me about ten years to understand what was going on. I'm still trying to understand my brain injury better. Headway is helping me with that – to learn more about my strengths and weaknesses.'

'What about your childhood?' I ask.

'I'm still angry with my parents and maybe I will always be,' says Liah. 'The feeling of emptiness, and being afraid, of being abandoned – that will never go. It will haunt me, but I have no choice but to accept it.'

It's hard to know what to say to this. I can't argue with it. I can't pretend to know what it feels like to be her or how she might begin to let go of the burden of her past.

I ask her if she sometimes imagines talking to her mum.

'Lots of times,' she says. 'What I usually say is, "Don't ever talk to me again!"' She laughs at this. 'Even as much as I'm angry with her, I do still think about her when I'm in a difficult situation. I think she is where I got my strength from. She didn't give up quickly. One day I'm hoping I will meet her again and just show her that I'm still here.'

I ask her about the future.

'This sounds so wrong,' she says after a moment. 'I haven't said it before, but to be honest I don't know anything apart from pain.' Her voice is steady now, though there are tears in her eyes. 'Maybe my life will change, but I don't think it will ever be the way I want it to be.'

According to an Amnesty International report, the third-largest group of people attempting to cross the Mediterranean into Europe in 2015 – after Syrians and Afghans – were Eritreans. It cites a UN estimate that at the end of 2014, 5,000 people were leaving Eritrea every month. As well as fleeing ongoing political and religious persecution, many of these people, the report says, are escaping Eritrea's system of 'indefinite national service' under which people as young as sixteen are conscripted for military training.

Though the official mandate is for eighteen months of duty, in reality the system channels conscripts into open-ended state indenture, paying poverty wages for agricultural work, construction, civil service and other 'patriotic duties'. Many people conscripted up to twenty years ago are still serving today, says the report, seeing their families infrequently and having little hope of escape. Deserters, including children, are imprisoned in inhumane conditions, 'often underground or in shipping containers', and 'risk torture or other ill-treatment'.

Of 14,000 people who graduated from military training in July 2016, the report says, '48% were women who experienced particularly harsh treatment, including sexual enslavement, torture and other sexual abuse'.

Perhaps Liah's loved ones were aware of what would happen to her if she stayed. Perhaps, with this knowledge in mind, it becomes easier to forgive them for abandoning her in a foreign country as an adolescent. The challenges that have faced her here in the UK surely pale in comparison to what she would have suffered in Eritrea. And, as Liah points out, at least here she stood a chance of receiving effective treatment for her HIV.

Liah says the Red Cross tried to find her mother back in 2004 but to no avail. It's impossible to say what has become of her since her arrest. The indications from Amnesty are not promising.

Is Liah asking too much? Is it simply unreasonable of her to want to live in a place that is both accessible and safe, a place that minimizes her reliance on others without at the same time isolating her from contact; a place that supports her physical agency without depriving her of opportunities to grow intellectually and emotionally or exposing her to the risk of assault or neglect?

There is a parallel between acquired disability and forced migration. In both cases – the sick patient and the desperate refugee – it is considered an intrinsic kindness to keep someone alive. But is this enough? If a child arrives with no family, no connections, no money, what is the least they should be offered once saved? And is it a forgivable cruelty, an excusable corollary of arguably limited resources, unrelentingly to revisit that orphan's homelessness, powerlessness, lovelessness upon them for the rest of their life?

It isn't the council's fault that Liah was born with HIV or that she contracted the PML that disabled her. It isn't the council's fault that there is a lack of accessible housing in London or that central government has cut the council's funding by 30 per cent in the last six years. It is, however, the council's responsibility to keep Liah safe and well – because she has nobody else.

It is a special condition of Liah's to be utterly dependent on the state. Not only to be without her own financial resources but to be unable physically to change her circumstances, to open the door and walk away. Perhaps when we picture the state as an entity that protects from harm the most vulnerable citizens within its reach, we don't do so with someone quite as vulnerable as Liah in mind. A failure of imagination, then.

'I went climbing with Bryn and a group of other Headway members,' Liah tells me. 'The wall I go on isn't quite vertical so I don't have to hold myself up totally, but it's still hard for me. I have to really concentrate to control my ataxia, my shaking. I've been twice before and

I managed to go up OK, but this time when I got halfway up the wall I got stuck. I couldn't go on and I couldn't go back. And then suddenly everything just flashed right in front of me – everything that's happened from the age of thirteen until now – and my legs wouldn't move. I came down on the rope and all I wanted to do was go outside to calm down, but the rope wouldn't come off. That's when I totally lost it.'

I picture Liah at the foot of the wall, racked with tears, furious, unable to untie the knot at her waist.

'It's the feeling of when you're trying to do something but you can't do it, no matter what you do, the frustration. That's how my life is. I'm stuck in one place and can't move anywhere. What do I do now? Do I give up? Do I carry on? I don't want to give up. The only way I can give up is – it sounds crazy when I say it – but the only way I can give up is actually dying. I've been stuck for so long. How do I end this? There's no end apart from just dying. But still I don't want to, so what do I do?

'When I got the rope off I went outside with Bryn. After I calmed down I came back in and carried on. I'm not going to let my emotions get to me. I'm not going to give up. One day I'm going to be the person who's helping someone.'

★

Tuesday 8 November.

> Hello Ben. Just got a call from Queen Square. They have moved my 6 January appointment to 19 November.
>
> I suspect that the new scans have confirmed my suspicions of significant further growth of the cyst.

> I suspect the surgeons at Queen Square will want to insert a shunt as quickly as possible.
>
> The other surgeon told me that a shunt is just a prophylactic. Apparently despite the shunt the cyst will eventually have to be removed.

None of this stacks up. The January appointment – the one they've moved – was to see a sleep specialist about the fatigue, nothing to do with the cyst. It's as though I'm watching the process of confabulation in action. Hospital letters are always ambiguous, pro-forma, full of blanks. When one comes through the door, Matthew immediately wants to know why it's been sent. Because he's smart, he can work out any number of explanations, but because he's amnesic those explanations are prone to being works of fiction coloured by anxiety. In this case he's not only mistaken the purpose of the appointment being re-scheduled, he's also imported an entire explanatory narrative that supports his worst fears.

Just a prophylactic. I wonder where he got this phrase. It sounds like one of his own. It's an amazing work of ellipsis, a neat little linguistic gloss, superficially truthful but obscuring a library's worth of subtle and contradictory information.

I text him back, for the record as much as anything, suggesting that a prophylactic that gives him ten to twenty years of life free of hydrocephalus and no further cognitive impairment might be a worthwhile investment. I don't wait for a reply. I ask him if he has spoken to his dad. He says not yet. He says Ayo is getting married soon. He wants to save his family the stress of what is happening to him at the moment. Then he tells me he's been weight training. It's been good for his mood, he says. 'Still very fatigued but happier.' He thinks I should give it a try. Ten minutes later he texts again:

> What was I supposed to speak to my dad about?

Thursday 10 November.

> Just spoke to the hospital. They have already scheduled the cyst removal for the 27th January 2017.
>
> They suddenly seem to be in a hurry.
>
> I guess my presumption of the cyst growing again over the last couple of months is somewhat valid.

> The surgery is at 07:00. That is very early in the morning. I will have to book a cab I suppose.

I compose a long text, pointing out the circularity of what's happening. I explain to him that the only person in a hurry is him. I say that the cyst hasn't grown in the last two months, he is confabulating this in response to a letter that came through the door – a letter that has been sent because he himself has elected to have the surgery. I tell him that he elected to have the surgery because he thinks it will make him better but that it won't. I tell him his sister was there at the appointment when he agreed to the surgery, but she's only going along with it because she doesn't know there is another, safer option. She doesn't know because he hasn't told her.

I wait ten seconds. I delete the text and write another one:

Hey Matthew. Thanks for keeping me posted. It sounds like you've decided to go ahead with cyst removal. Do you think it would be wise to talk to your dad soon? Do you plan to tell him about the shunt option?

Ben, the guys at my hospital think the shunt is a delaying tactic.

I have spoken to my dad. He feels that the removal is preferable.

Of course he does. I picture the conversation. 'Just a prophylactic,' says Matthew. 'Delaying tactic. Cyst will have to come out eventually.' I have never met Matthew's father. I have no idea what kind of person he is. He and the rest of the family are a blank somewhere far away in a country I have never visited. Not for the first time I picture myself calling them. But that's not how it works.

After some false starts I manage to get through to the neurosurgery secretary. I ask if I can book a follow-up appointment with the surgeon offering to remove Matthew's cyst, whose name, I have learned, is Mr Da Rocha. She says things are very booked up. She will call me back.

★

Thursday 24 November.

Hello Ben. Was reviewing the letter about the surgery with Ernest. Apparently I need to be escorted to the hospital on the day.

Will have to tell Ayo about the exact date then.

Or if you are able to help on the day that might be useful.

Thanks. Sorry to put you in this position.

I'm expecting a call about the new clinic apt with Mr Da Rocha. If you want me to come on the day of the surgery I will. But let's see what happens at the next clinic first, eh?

OK. What do you think having the next clinic will achieve precisely?

We've been through this, but I repeat it all the same. I tell him I want to ask why removal is preferable to having a shunt, why the surgeon thinks he can remove the cyst completely given the failure last time, why he thinks he can do it without causing further cognitive impairment, whether he's operating on the basis that Matthew has elected to have the surgery and if so does he feel he's made an adequate assessment of Matthew's understanding of the risks involved and the other available options. I say I also want to ask if the surgeon can account for the fact that his colleague at Queen Square is contradicting his advice. Matthew texts back:

> Seems more than fair.
>
> But having to deal with all of this is really exhausting.

> I know. I'm sorry.

★

Friday 25 November. The secretary calls saying that, luckily, there has been a cancellation. There is a slot open next Monday. I check with Matthew that he's free and call back to confirm.

I text Matthew to ask if he will bring Ayo.

> Not sure if that is a good idea. It exposes her to more bad news.

★

Monday 28 November. I can feel my hands trembling slightly as Matthew and I settle on the yellow plastic chairs in the little assessment room. I'm tense because I know this meeting is happening too late. The idea of the surgery now has momentum, so I'm already at a disadvantage, working against a solidifying future. But I'm also nervous because of the feeling of mistrust I've developed for this department. The consultants have been inconsistent, muddled, vague. And on some level I'm concerned they are offering Matthew something they shouldn't. I am, in a certain respect, already in conflict with the man we are here to meet.

Mr Da Rocha has a soft face and a mild accent. He looks a little tired. It's the end of the day. And, as though he too is aware of the tension behind our meeting, he shifts awkwardly at the sight of my audio recorder. It's already switched on. I ask him if he minds.

'I don't mind,' he says, but there's doubt in his voice. 'There are printed letters,' he says.

'I know,' I say, 'but there is a lot of information that needs to be understood in order to make the right decision.' I'm not sure why it should be a problem. Nobody else has raised an eyebrow. Surely neurosurgeons must encounter this all the time, working with patients who have memory impairments.

'Sure,' he says. 'OK. Just for my understanding, did someone appoint you or . . . ?'

Matthew steps in. 'No. I've been at Headway for quite a while, since I had my brain injury, and I've been supported by them as an organization regularly – with respect to benefits and other help.'

'I don't need to see any paperwork, do I?' says Mr Da Rocha. 'Because I've never come across this before. I mean on the ward, yes, but not at a clinic appointment.'

I'm not sure what he means. 'Do you want to see my ID?' I ask, reaching for my wallet.

'I don't want to,' he says, turning to Matthew. 'If you're happy?'

'It's fine,' says Matthew.

At this Mr Da Rocha seems to relent. 'We are all doing this for you,' he says.

He turns to his computer. 'So your last scan was in June,' he says, 'right?'

'Yep,' says Matthew.

'You had one at Queen Square more recently,' I say.

'Really?' says Mr Da Rocha and it's immediately obvious that he didn't know about the other consultations, that Matthew didn't mention them last time they met. 'And why was that? Was it urgent?'

'Ah, no,' says Matthew, 'because I'd seen them as well, with respect to my tumour.'

'It's not a tumour,' says Mr Da Rocha, crisply. 'It's a cyst. A benign thing.' He seems irritated. 'Who did you see?'

'Mr Khoury,' says Matthew. 'And he was suggesting that a shunt would be a good option.'

'I think this is a very bad idea,' says Mr Da Rocha, 'seeing two different units, two different surgeons, because everyone will tell you a different thing. Everyone specializes in a different thing. Do you have a letter from Samir? I know Samir.'

Samir is Mr Khoury's first name. I can't tell from Mr Da Rocha's tone what he thinks of Mr Khoury. I can't tell if it's good or bad that they know each other.

'On me?' says Matthew. 'No.'

'But you have a letter at home?'

'Yes,' says Matthew.

I don't know why the letter matters. Would we invent the consultations with Mr Khoury? What would a letter prove? I explain that I've raised the possibility with Matthew of choosing one or other department to work with, but that this hasn't happened yet. I say that I'm concerned that the current situation is causing some mixed messages and that it's not good for Matthew. 'Maybe it's not good for you either?' I hazard.

'It's not great for us,' says Mr Da Rocha. 'We don't know what was discussed, we don't know what was agreed. We all have different experiences.' He has turned back to his monitor and is clicking through the scans again. 'I also don't know if my colleagues there have seen all the previous scans.'

'They've seen scans since 2008,' I say, 'I think.'

'When was your operation?' Mr Da Rocha asks.

'2005,' says Matthew.

'So this was your scan from 2016,' says Mr Da Rocha, showing us the all-too-familiar greyscale image of the inside of Matthew's head. 'This is your scan from 2008.'

'Right,' says Matthew.

'I'm sure we discussed them last time as well,' says Mr Da Rocha. His annoyance is still near the surface. He begins to revise what he knows, a repetition of what we've heard a hundred times. 'This is a picture of your brain from the side. This is the cyst. It's in an area called the third ventricle.' I suppose it makes sense to assume we know nothing. I suppose it's good revision for Matthew. 'In 2008 this cyst was about ten millimetres,' he says. 'Now it's much bigger. It's about seventeen, I'd say. We can measure it.'

He clicks his mouse at the image a few times, drawing a line that cuts the pale circle of the cyst in half across its diameter, but he seems to get bored of that idea and instead turns back to Matthew once more. 'So there is an increase in size over the course of several years,' he says, 'and there are risks if we leave it untreated: drop attacks, sudden death or developing acute hydrocephalus. Right now you don't have any symptoms of headaches or vomiting, do you?'

'No,' says Matthew.

'So putting a shunt in would be a preventative type of operation,' says Mr Da Rocha. 'But a shunt does not address the colloid cyst, it only addresses the hydrocephalus. Sometimes we see small cysts causing these problems of drop attacks or sudden death,' he says again, 'even small cysts that don't cause hydrocephalus, if that makes sense.'

It doesn't make sense. Mr Khoury has spent the whole summer telling us that the hydrocephalus is the only way that the cyst can do any harm and that the cyst could only be dangerous once it grows big enough to cause a blockage. The other consultants, Mr Da Rocha's own colleagues, here at this hospital, have spent many years saying the same thing.

'Obviously your case is a bit more complicated because you've had an operation in the past and there have been residual neurological deficits from that intervention, I guess.'

It's almost a question but not quite. It's more of an inference, a supposition. Matthew is silent. I take my cue.

'My concern is around the risk associated with repeat surgery,' I say. 'Mr Khoury is suggesting that a shunt would represent the possibility of deferring any further intervention and that it would be lower risk than removing the cyst.'

'The shunt itself is lower risk than removing the cyst,' says Mr Da Rocha, 'absolutely. But what would be the aim of deferring the operation – to operate in the future or never to operate?'

'Potentially never, is his position,' I say, 'I think.' It's weird to be speaking for a neurosurgeon. It's weird to be confronting another neurosurgeon with a contradiction to his advice. 'But I don't want to necessarily cause you to have to defend your position,' I say, trying to be polite.

'I have no position to defend,' says Mr Da Rocha. 'Someone has referred you to me because I operate on a lot of these patients. In my mind it's very clear what needs to happen and I'm trying to explain it to you.' He turns to Matthew. 'You have a large cyst. The cyst is growing. It's a bit more complicated because you had a procedure in the past and because you've been affected in terms of memory or . . . I don't know if you have any cognitive issues or neuropsychology issues' – again, the almost-question is left hanging – 'but in your age group I would recommend that this is treated. You're twenty-nine, you're not sixty-nine.'

'Thirty-eight,' Matthew says.

'Yes, thirty-eight, sorry,' Mr Da Rocha says, but seems not to register any impact his miscalculation may have. 'So you're young and this is still growing.'

I try another tack. I tell him about our meeting with Mr Hau, about how he said that, though he couldn't remember the specifics, he believed they would have tried to remove the cyst. I tell him that, on this basis, I'm concerned that whatever stopped them completing the job last time would still be a problem on a second attempt. 'Do you think that's a reasonable concern?' I ask him.

'It is a reasonable concern,' he says, 'yes.'

'Is there anything that's changed since then that would make it more likely that you could remove it successfully this time?'

'Well, I wasn't there at the previous operation,' says Mr Da Rocha, 'so I don't know what problems they encountered, if they encountered any problems. I don't know what their strategy was. So I don't know how to answer to this particular concern.'

'Maybe you could help us understand what your strategy would be this time,' I say, 'your approach?'

'Yes, of course. There are several ways to operate on a colloid cyst. One is what they did in the past with a craniotomy.' He shows us the old surgical track on the scans as well as a smaller track on the left side from the external ventricular drain that was put in. It's extraordinary how, each time we look at the scans, some further damage is pointed out.

His favoured approach, he explains, would be to go through on the left side this time. 'You can see the cyst facing towards the left now,' he says, 'going through the foramen on that side.'

He's right. In the slice shown on the screen the cyst is shaped slightly like a teardrop, bulging to the left.

He says he would make a single hole in the cranium, rather than taking an entire section away, as happened last time, and would go through the existing track caused by the drain that was inserted back in 2005. And he would use an endoscope in order to keep the damage to a minimum.

'With the endoscope we can take a look up-close. We have instruments that go through the endoscope shaft, so it's a different tool, a different technique than last time. I'm not trying to say that one technique or approach is better than the other one, but it is well known nowadays that the endoscope is very good kit in experienced hands.'

'OK,' I say. 'If you go from the other side, what would the risks to the other fornix be?'

'There's always a risk of memory problems. I'm pretty sure I mentioned last time that we can make you worse with the operation in terms of memory or in terms of fine neuropsychological assessment. There are other risks like bleeding, infection, fluid leak; there is a small risk of stroke and a small risk of death with these operations. There's a small risk of recurrence.'

'So even assuming the cyst is removed successfully,' I say, 'are you able to give any kind of estimate of the risks of further cognitive impairment?'

'In terms of a percentage, you mean?' asks Mr Da Rocha.

'Whatever you choose,' I say.

'No, it's very hard to tell.'

'I see,' I say. 'If I'm right in my understanding, then with the colloid cyst there are particular risks to the fornix?'

'There are particular risks,' he says, 'yes, because you dissect a bit more than in more routine hydrocephalus operations. But there are less risks than when you're doing an intra-ventricular tumour.'

It's hard to tell if the issue here is really so complex as Mr Da Rocha is making it seem. All I want to know is: on balance, is Mr Khoury right? Maybe it's a stupid question.

'So if Matthew had a shunt, are you saying you think that won't be enough?'

He answers with another question: 'How did he suggest to do that? A single shunt with a perforation between the ventricles?'

'I don't know,' I say.

'Because if he's going to put an endoscope in and do a perforation in the middle we might as well put an endoscope in and remove the colloid cyst.'

'I see,' I say, 'because that would carry similar risks, would it?'

'Yes,' says Mr Da Rocha, and qualifies himself: 'Although the risks are very, very low with the perforation, in fact.'

'Lower than trying to remove the cyst?'

'Oh yes, absolutely,' he says. 'Much lower.' I can't tell how much of this Matthew is taking on board. It's using all of my concentration just to follow what Mr Da Rocha is saying. It's starting to feel very much like he's thinking on his feet, like this might be the first time he's followed this line of questioning. Or, worse, as though he's in conflict with himself, as though he has committed himself to the idea that cyst removal is the best option and can't back down despite the simple fact that his argument doesn't add up.

'I mean, we don't disagree with Mr Khoury,' he says. I don't know who he means by 'we'. 'The shunt is a smaller operation with smaller risks, but the risk from an untreated colloid cyst that is about seventeen millimetres and growing is significant.'

'Right,' I say. 'So, aside from hydrocephalus, can you explain what harm is done by the untreated cyst?'

'That's very difficult,' says Mr Da Rocha. 'There are all sorts of theories. Some people say that there is a sort of movement of the cyst, because it's hanging from the roof of the third ventricle and may cause a blockage.'

'But again,' I say, 'that would be to do with increased pressure?'

'Potentially,' says Mr Da Rocha. 'We don't know the mechanism. Or at least not that I'm aware of. I mean, if that's the case we would treat every colloid cyst with a shunt. By far the gold standard is to resect the colloid cyst.'

'I see,' I say. 'It's only difficult because that's not the message we've been given by Mr Khoury.'

I don't know what I'm hoping for. Maybe that, rather than simply trying to cajole us, or win the argument, Mr Da Rocha could join us in trying to work out the best answer to this life-and-death conundrum, could work with us, as a collaborator, attempting to view the situation from Matthew's perspective. Maybe I just want him to listen. But that doesn't seem to be on the cards. 'Mr Khoury is saying that cyst removal would be very risky,' I continue.

'Why?' Mr Da Rocha asks.

'I think in terms of cognitive impairment,' I say. 'He's saying that a shunt would be a very low-risk way of managing the hydrocephalus.'

Mr Da Rocha says nothing to this, just looks at us and nods.

I move on to another line of enquiry. 'Again,' I say, 'just for the record, because this is something Matthew has been confused about, if the cyst is taken away is it likely to have any positive impact on his impairments around memory or fatigue or other symptoms?'

'Most likely not. I don't think we can hope for that.'

'OK,' I say, wanting to make sure Matthew has heard this. He is silent, gazing levelly at Mr Da Rocha. I'm sure this is way too much information for him. I'm sure he's switched off. 'I think in the past that's something Matthew has hoped for.'

I look from Mr Da Rocha to Matthew and realize how far I am from having an understanding of what's in either of their minds.

'Does the hospital offer any support around this kind of decision-making,' I ask, 'beyond the consultations with the surgeons?'

'What do you mean?' says Mr Da Rocha. 'Like a second opinion?'

'I mean outside of this room. If there were a patient whose ability to hold on to all of the necessary information is impaired, is that something the hospital can offer assistance with?'

'I'm sure it is,' says Mr Da Rocha. 'I can ask the legal services.' And now it appears that something comes into his mind for the first time: 'Does Matthew have . . . He's not under the Mental Capacity Act, is he?'

'What do you mean, not under it?' I ask.

'Has his mental capacity been assessed properly?'

On the one hand, this is exactly the question I've been hoping Mr Da Rocha will consider. On the other, his wording suggests that, like many doctors, he hasn't had training on the Mental Capacity Act. The Act stipulates that capacity can't be assessed 'globally' as a property the person either does or doesn't possess, in the way that Mr Da Rocha's wording implies. Instead, capacity must be assessed with reference to any given decision whose significance warrants it, on a case-by-case basis.

'I would suggest that an assessment should really be performed,' I say. 'Though Matthew presents extremely well I'm not entirely confident that he has the capacity to make this decision without support.'

Matthew makes a noise: 'Ummm.'

'Who is at home with you?' asks Mr Da Rocha.

'I live alone,' Matthew replies.

'And do you cope on a daily basis?'

'Yes,' says Matthew. 'I'm really untidy but I think that's a depressive problem.'

Mr Da Rocha nods slowly. 'I think he understands the implications,' he says, almost to himself. And then: 'It's a serious operation, it's not without risk. I can understand why we have these discussions where we think about it. I can understand why you're seeing someone else and that's absolutely fine. There are many options here and every option has advantages and disadvantages.' It's a pronounced change of tone from the beginning of the meeting, when the idea of another surgeon being involved seemed to provoke nothing but annoyance.

I can see that Matthew is itching. 'I beg your pardon,' he says. 'From my rational understanding the problem boils down to a question of which surgery you want to do first. Have the shunt inserted and wait a couple of years or deal with the cyst now before it becomes too difficult. It's simply a case of ordering.'

'It's not entirely like this,' says Mr Da Rocha. 'It's not a case of order, because Mr Khoury has suggested a shunt-only operation where you may never need the cyst removed. That's the alternative.'

'I'd rather be rid of the cyst, personally,' says Matthew. 'It's a risk I'd be willing to take.' It's as though he can't hear what's being said.

'Do you want me to see your family again?' asks Mr Da Rocha, perhaps, finally, responding to the possibility that Matthew's word shouldn't just be flatly accepted without further consideration.

'My parents are in Nigeria,' says Matthew. 'I've spoken to my dad about it and he's fine.'

'And they're aware that there is another option,' says Mr Da Rocha, 'with the shunt and everything, right?'

'I've mentioned that to my dad,' says Matthew, 'but I think I've told him of the risks, that sometimes it might need to be replaced if it gets blocked.'

'Yes,' says Mr Da Rocha, 'but in your case you're at high risk that you will need the shunt eventually. Either right after surgery or sometime in the future.'

This is new information. 'Sometime in the future . . . ?' I say.

'I don't know,' says Mr Da Rocha. 'Hard to say.'

I turn to Matthew. 'My concern is that, though we've been through these conversations repeatedly, and though you have talked to your family about it, the effect of the confabulation and the memory loss and your own instinct to be rid of the cyst – these things might affect the kind of information you're sharing with your dad. I'm concerned that you may be weighting the descriptions for him in a way that represents the shunt as a delaying tactic and might not perhaps share the degree of risk concerned with the cyst removal.'

'Right,' says Matthew. 'But still, at some point the cyst would have to come out, right?' He turns to Mr Da Rocha. 'Because if it grows into the fornix then it becomes inoperable?'

Mr Da Rocha frowns. 'No,' he says haltingly, 'it's not a tumour that we would deem as inoperable. I've operated on bigger colloid cysts.'

Matthew nods. 'I'm fine with the cyst removal,' he says. 'It's a risk I'd be willing to take.'

'I'll have a chat with the legal services,' says Mr Da Rocha, 'see what they suggest. If they suggest an assessment by a member of our psychiatric team would you be happy to do that?'

'As long as it doesn't disturb the surgery on the day,' says Matthew.

'Because, as far as I'm concerned, I have a date for the surgery and I'm sticking to it.'

We are running out of things to talk about.

'OK,' says Mr Da Rocha. 'Fine. Good. We'll proceed as planned and we'll get an assessment done in the meantime.'

Matthew and I walk east, away from the hospital, under a night sky. Yellow lights move past us along the road. It's bitterly cold. I ask him what he thinks. He lets out a breath between his lips.

'Either way I'm screwed,' he says.

'Shit,' I say. 'There you go again.'

'What do you mean?'

'You're talking like you don't have a choice.'

He shakes his head, sighs again. 'The cyst has got to come out.'

It's as though we're in a dead end together, saying the same things again and again, neither of us able to understand the other, waiting for someone to come and rescue us, someone who knows everything, can see it all from above, and will swoop down and tell us what to do. An angel. In a red helicopter.

'Do you think I'm being rational about this?' Matthew asks me as we cross a side street. 'Or fatalistic?'

'Fatalistic,' I say. 'That's the word.'

He nods. 'Why can't you put your faith in God?' he says. I don't know if he's joking or being deadly serious. There's no frown and no laugh. 'If you put your faith in God things work out better.'

★

The following day, sitting at my desk, I notice I am having some strong feelings. Anxiety. Fear. Loneliness.

I talk to my colleague Anya, our OT and the staff member most familiar with the Mental Capacity Act. She says I'm doing the right things. She offers to help me draw up a summary of the information we have so far, so that Matthew can have it all in front of him at once, to help him balance out the pros and cons.

I talk to Nora. When I describe the operation being offered she claps her hands to either side of her face. 'Shit,' she says. 'He's going to give himself another brain injury.' I talk her through the plan and she says to keep her in the loop.

I send Mr Da Rocha an email repeating what I said about the need for a mental capacity assessment. I cc Anya, Nora and Matthew on the email.

Matthew texts me shortly after.

> Ben I think you should do the following:
> 1. Read up on what it feels like to live with a colloid cyst
>
> 2. What it feels like to live with a ventricular shunt system
>
> I have no other choice. The cyst has to come out.

> And please don't pull a psychology crap of lack of mental soundness on me. I am as sound as they come. I am making a rational choice based on my symptoms.
>
> Living with persistently achy bones and muscles is not at all pleasant.
>
> Let this be alright!

The texts illustrate the problem perfectly. He's going back and back to the delusional hope that removing the cyst will make him better. My email has annoyed him, but that's a price I'm willing to pay if it buys us some time. That's really what it's about: making the surgeon take a step backwards, buying some time.

The next day Matthew sends another text to similar effect, angry with me for questioning the research he's done on the Internet. He says the Internet is 'currently the most used source of information on the planet'. Later he sends another one with an apologetic tone.

> Sorry to have you in this situation Ben.
>
> Really sorry.
>
> It is not fair on you to be in this position.

I tell him not to worry.

Da Rocha emails back, saying he has spoken to his team and the legal department at the hospital. He says he plans to book a neuro-psychology assessment for Matthew. This isn't the same thing as a mental capacity assessment, but it's a start. He also says he'll ask for a second opinion from another surgeon in the trust. I reply, telling him I'm not sure a third opinion is really what Matthew needs. I tell him that, ideally, I'd like to see the department here collaborate with Queen Square towards a unified recommendation. I have no idea how realistic this is. I tell him I'll contact Queen Square and ask them to share their neuropsychology assessment with him.

Much of the week is taken up with other Headway business: inter-viewing applicants for a staff vacancy, meeting with the CEO and board members about future development, negotiating staff pay scales. But all the while, part of my mind is thinking about Matthew. I can feel him there in the background, in the dark street, the cul-de-sac we have walked into together. He hasn't been at the centre this week and I can guess why: he isn't sleeping.

On the Thursday evening I cycle over to Stratford for the opening evening of Headway's first public art exhibition. I've been asked to give a speech. Standing in front of the small crowd of supporters who have turned out, I quote an American painter called Robert Henri: 'I paint for the sole purpose of magnifying the privilege of being alive.' I hadn't heard of Henri before, but it's that word, 'privilege', that made me pick him out. Is being alive an inherent privilege? I think of the time Danny told me: *If anything like that should ever happen again, switch the machine off.* I think of Matthew, of what he's going through right now.

As I make my way home that night he texts me:

> It's funny how everyone I ask for advice just seems to speak without really offering much in terms of definite direction.
>
> It all seems to boil down to 'it's your problem mate, not mine.'
>
> That is understandable, given the circumstance.
>
> But thanks for all your help.

I read the text several times. Once again he's seen right to the heart of the problem. The surgeons are treating him like a customer, presenting him with a choice between options that purport to be equivalent when, in fact, they are nothing of the sort. It's a consumer model that is totally out of place in the context of life-and-death medical care. There is far too much specialist knowledge involved for it to work. And it leaves Matthew, a man already coping with multiple, complex health challenges, in the position of having to choose his fate on an inevitably partial view of the facts.

I sit down and draw up the table Anya and I discussed: the pros and cons of the two procedures being offered, what the two surgeons have said about risks and benefits. I send the table to both Mr Da Rocha and

Mr Khoury and ask if they would kindly review it and send me any corrections. I want it to be accurate.

Then I set about transcribing the audio from the appointment with Mr Da Rocha. As I type I find myself listening more and more closely to his choice of words.

'I wasn't there at the previous operation,' he says, 'so I don't know what problems they encountered . . . I don't know what their strategy was.' It's a focus on technique rather than physiology. If they'd gone about it in the right way, they would have been successful, that's the implication.

'If it's something like this we usually go back in and operate . . . It's not unheard of to re-operate on a colloid cyst . . . It is well known nowadays that the endoscope is very good kit in experienced hands.'

We: something collective. Not just the responsibility of one person.

It's not unheard of: an appeal to external authority, to shared knowledge, to convention.

It is well known: convention again.

Nowadays: the latest knowledge. If you don't know this, maybe you're behind the times.

Very good kit: technology, expensive stuff, for the boys.

Experienced hands: technique, skill, steadiness. Whose hands? His hands.

I hear my own voice: 'Are you able to explain, with the cyst, beyond hydrocephalus, what the mechanism of harm is?'

'We're still looking for that mechanism in the literature,' he replies.

In the literature. I picture people reading books. Where is the mechanism?

'I'm sure that you might have googled a little bit, but there are all sorts of theories of why it happens,' he says. 'Some people say that there is a sort of movement of the cyst, because it's hanging from the roof of the third ventricle and may cause a blockage . . .'

'But again,' I say, 'that would be to do with increased pressure?' I'm pressing him on this point. I want him to say categorically that there is another mechanism or there isn't. Or at least make a case for how there could be.

'Potentially,' says Mr Da Rocha. 'We don't know the mechanism. Or at least not that I'm aware of.' And then: 'I mean, if that's the case we would treat every colloid cyst with a shunt.'

There is an utterance missing, a thought that occurred to him but that he didn't voice: *Maybe hydrocephalus is the only mechanism of harm.* But this causes a short circuit. He can't accept the idea that surgeons would be removing these cysts if it weren't necessary. Then, almost to acknowledge the failure in his reasoning, he says of the shunt: 'And it is an option. It is an option . . .'

Towards the end of the discussion I notice that I begin openly questioning Mr Da Rocha's use of language, repeating his words back to him, boxing him in. In response he begins to repeat the words himself so that, at one point, the dialogue becomes like a Beckett play, breaking down into echoing fragments, the voices getting slower and quieter as we grapple with the collapse of our communication.

'. . . By far the gold standard is to resect the colloid cyst,' says Mr Da Rocha. 'It is the gold standard.'

'Gold standard,' I say, 'what does that mean?'

'The gold standard,' he says. 'The standard operation. The best option.'

'Best in terms of what?'

'In terms of everything,' he says. 'The mainstay of treatment.'

'The mainstay.'

Gold standard: like a seal of approval, I think, like precious metal, top prize, quality mark, like milk or safety glass. *Mainstay*: convention, what everybody does. We all do it. There must be a reason if we're all doing it.

It's not clear to me why I'm obsessing over his language like this, trying to find fault. Somehow we have been cast as adversaries instead of friends. He's annoyed at being questioned, I'm angered by his annoyance, and by the implacability of the system he represents. My thoughts are overtaking me.

I hear myself ask if it's possible for the hospital to support Matthew any further with the decision.

'I'm sure it is,' he says, 'I can ask the legal services.'

'The legal services.' I say. 'How would we do that?'

And here his voice becomes so quiet I can barely make it out on the recording: 'I could contact them. I could contact them.'

I remember in a flash that I still have Matthew's hospital notes from his admission in 2005. I dig them out and leaf through them until I find a consent form for the operation, signed by Matthew. It's been filled out by hand. Under 'Responsible health professional' it says 'Hau'. Under 'Name of proposed procedure or intervention', it says 'Craniotomy for excision of 3rd ventricle colloid cyst +/- bilateral ventricular shunt'.

This is proof that they did indeed try to remove the cyst the first time. I don't know why I didn't think to look for this before. I scan it and send it to both Matthew and Mr Da Rocha.

I spend an hour on the phone with Bryan, the neuropsychologist at Queen Square. He seems concerned that Mr Da Rocha hasn't assessed Matthew's mental capacity. He agrees that this should be a priority. But he also helps me see that I have to limit my involvement in the quandary somehow. It has to be Matthew's decision, he says. And assuming Matthew has capacity, he must be free to make a choice that seems irrational or ill-advised or that might appear, from my point of view, to be against his own best interests. I know he's right. This is one of the central tenets of the Mental Capacity Act: if someone is shown to have capacity, then they can make any decision they like.

Bryan says I need to get Matthew's family more closely involved. I need to share what information I have with them. They are the ones who are best placed to help Matthew in deciding what to do. Apart from anything else, he says, I could be putting myself at risk if I argue too strongly one way or another. 'What if you manage to talk him out of having the cyst removed,' he says, 'and then he gets really sick or dies and then his family sue you?'

He says that maybe Matthew's mental health is affecting his thinking, 'But these things affect all of us. You can say that what he's doing isn't rational and it's frustrating for you to see it happening, but we're all irrational. And we don't know what it's like for him living with the cyst.'

Neither of the surgeons has responded to my request for them to look at the decision table I'd drawn up for Matthew. Bryan kindly agrees to take a look himself, 'Though I'm not a surgeon,' he says.

'I know,' I say, 'but you're the only health professional involved who's made the time to talk to me on the phone.'

2017

Christmas passes quietly. I'm left alone for a few days, during which I manage to do very little. A few days later I travel up to Scotland with friends, to the small island of Eigg.

On New Year's Day I join a walk up the volcanic plug in the middle of the island. From the top we can see the ocean in all directions. A mile out at sea there is both rain and sun, separated by empty air, like yesterday and tomorrow, beating into the water. The rock is so sheer as to create the impression of being detached, somehow free-floating. A rainbow hovers next to it, its vault above us, its sides curving into the ground a thousand yards below, piercing the gorse at a point just before it becomes a full circle. I close my eyes and see wet rock, thick bracken stems stuttering under my hand.

A shower passes, rain clicking against my hood. A pair of ravens circle up and around the rock, pass through the steady rainbow, and dive again.

It occurs to me that I have been living for some weeks now somehow *inside* my thoughts rather than with them. I can feel the strain I have been putting my mind under. It won't do me any good. It's impossible to say what good, if any, it can do Matthew.

But I do have choices. Another perspective is possible. I can choose between my roles. I can choose to be Matthew's friend and to stay exposed to all this danger, all this fear, or I can choose to revert to something safer, to go back to being a professional.

It's clear that I should do as Bryan suggests. Once he's had a look at the table I should show it to Matthew and ask his permission to share it with his family. And then I should step back.

★

Back at work I arrange for Matthew to see one of Headway's psychotherapists, Gwen. Matthew seems happy to go along with it, but I sense it's mainly to keep me happy. 'It's just so that I know I've done my job properly,' I say. 'So I can show someone else has spoken to you on the record.'

A week later Matthew texts me to say a date for surgery has been confirmed by letter: Wednesday 8 February. Less than two weeks away. The letter says he needs to be accompanied by a responsible adult. He asks if I will go with him. I say yes.

> You are still thinking that this is a very bad idea, aren't you?

> It doesn't matter what I think – only you know what's best for you.

> Really?

> Well . . . think about it from my perspective. If I discourage you from having the operation and the cyst kills you 2 weeks later, then where do I stand? Equally, if I tell you to go for it and the operation is a botch, I'm in the same rather sad boat.

> I've tried to take the most empirical view I can – going with what the surgeons are saying but not just taking their word for anything . . . but I also know this isn't just about being reasonable. It's not science. It's your life and your mind. And you have to live with the cyst. I can't know what that feels like or what I would do in your position.

So I have to try and support you whatever you decide. Right?

Yes I understand. It is just a very bad and unfortunate circumstance. Thank you very much for all your help and support. Cannot have been easy. It is just life. But by historical standards it is a minor kerfuffle. No?

You mean compared to the 2nd World War?

Yup. Or living before modern medicine or 1st World War trench warfare. Or American slavery or any of the difficulties currently being experienced by people around the world.

Yeah. Compared to all those your situation is a cinch.

Cinch?

Sinch?

Sintsh?

Cinch:
1. Something easy to accomplish
2. A sure thing or a certainty

That's the one.

When I try to think about Matthew it's as though the future has become clouded now. After so much thinking, the situation suddenly won't admit any action of the mind. All that seems possible is to feel. It's harder for me to identify feelings, but I'm aware of something over the next few days. Walking to work, lying in the bath, cleaning the kitchen, there's a steady ache if I stay still a moment, behind the sounds of everything else.

*

Friday 3 February. I wake in the small hours full of doubt.

There is bias on both sides, I see that. The surgeons don't routinely deal with people disabled by their interventions. How survivors live and cope day to day is not their concern and they see so many deaths that survival is to them a decent outcome. You're alive? You can use your hands, or one hand? You can see? We did our job well.

In my work, however, all I see is disability, consequence, lives diverted or destroyed by brain injury. I'm hyper-vigilant to morbidity, to loss, to the hazards inherent in interfering with the contents of the skull.

*

Sunday 5 February. I've been in denial myself. Matthew has been saying it for months, but I haven't been able to hear it. He said it in the meeting with Da Rocha, repeated it many times. *I'd rather be rid of the cyst. The cyst has got to come out.* Gwen had confirmed it for me after the appointment with him:

'He's scared of the cyst, scared of dying. That's the biggest thing in his mind.'

I have been trying to defend Matthew against potential harm, to preserve him against an action that represents the risk of damaging who he is. But if I try to take away his choice now, today, I am robbing him of the very thing I am trying to protect: his will, his agency, his self. And for Matthew as much as anyone I've met, the ability to choose his own fate is what makes him who he is.

It's like this: defend a theoretical Matthew, a Matthew of the future who cannot ultimately be known, or defend the real Matthew, the living, breathing Matthew who stands in front of me, who is telling me what he wants to do with every fibre of his being.

However much I dread the action Matthew is about to take, all I can do is help him take it.

Tuesday 7 February, 12.50 p.m.

> How are you feeling?

Alright. My go-to model for this psychological state is to presume I am about to face the death penalty. What is to fear precisely? The process of dying or what comes after?

But I guess in the case of brain surgery, what comes after is the scary bit. Which makes the death penalty psychologically easier I suppose.

The irony.

> Don't worry. By the law of averages you've had more than your share of bad luck so the likelihood is that things will start to turn around after tomorrow. Also, bear in mind this is very different from last time – not an emergency, and everyone is much more prepared, so will go much smoother. It'll be like a holiday!

★

Wednesday 8 February. I cycle south and east through the dark of the pre-dawn. The temperature is just above freezing and the city is full of fog.

On my prior visits, the hospital has been bustling with visitors and staff but today the lobby is silent. I'm the only person in the lift. The building is so quiet I wonder if I'm in the right place. The doors all seem to be locked. Eventually I find my way into the neurosurgery ward and discover Matthew sitting next to Ayo in the visitors' room with a large holdall between his feet.

'Did you get any sleep?' I ask.

'No,' says Matthew. 'I wanted to be zoned out.' He's told me he has a phobia of needles. When he was hospitalized in 2005, he says, he wouldn't let them anaesthetize him. He's kept himself awake all night specifically in order to be extra tired today.

'Thanks for coming,' says Ayo. She's always polite but I never quite know what she thinks of me. She sits quietly next to Matthew.

There's one other patient in the room: a middle-aged man, with his wife and son. In the awkward silence it occurs to me that this is a little like catching a long-haul flight. You get up early, trek across the city tired and then sit in a grey room in your jacket with some strangers, waiting for something to happen.

Outside the window a dense fog has descended, obscuring all but the closest buildings.

A nurse puts tags around each of Matthew's wrists and checks his details. A while later a junior doctor in blue scrubs comes in to talk through the surgery one more time. We ask him how long it will take. He explains that there are three other operations ahead of Matthew's, scheduled for the morning. 'They're quite big surgeries,' he says, 'but Mr Da Rocha is quite a quick surgeon in the morning.'

Shortly after that, another nurse takes us to a room down the corridor and explains that, in all likelihood, it will be early evening before he goes into theatre. Matthew, utterly exhausted, lies down on the bed.

I go into work for a few hours and return at around 3 p.m. to find Matthew still on the bed, half asleep, Ayo sitting nearby, looking at her phone, and Ted, another friend of Matthew's, sitting next to the bed.

Matthew met Ted at a vocational rehab course he did some years ago. Ted has a brain injury too – from a fall. He points out that someone has drawn a black arrow on the left side of Matthew's forehead, pointing at the old scar from the last time he had surgery. He laughs gently. 'So they don't forget it's brain surgery they're doing.'

Somehow the subject of God comes up.

'Are you religious, Matthew?' asks Ted.

'Partly,' Matthew replies. 'I don't believe God is a sadomasochist. I don't believe he wants to punish us.'

'Do you believe in God, though?'

'Of course I do,' says Matthew. 'But it's not straightforward.'

What had he told Rayhana? God is a bucket of water.

A few minutes later the nurses arrive to take Matthew away. We all give him a hug and wish him luck. 'See you in a few hours,' I say.

I go home for a while to rest. I make dinner with Chris. Standing at the kitchen sink I try to think about the likely scenarios. Last time it seems like disorientation was the cause of a lot of problems after the surgery. If they damage the fornix again, Matthew might forget the most recent events, like going into hospital and why he's there. Is there something we can do to reassure him? What would that be? Will it help to see familiar faces? I can't imagine what else would help. I'm too tired to think.

I ask myself, how does it work? How are we, animals, selves, minds, possible? *How are we?* How is it at all that we persist and remain recognizable to ourselves? That we don't simply vanish, evaporate in the sunshine, implode into steam? It seems so much more likely that any given person should not exist or, existing, cease to, at any, every, moment. It's the being at all that's astonishing, and the continuing to be.

And now it seems to me that Matthew has vanished, become more a proposition than a person, something that exists only in theory and might or might not return. He has become an idea, a shade of himself in the hands of others.

Lying in the bath I fall asleep for a few minutes. Disappearing from myself I am momentarily in another place, warm and dark, where the only thing discernible is the sound of a voice talking steadily. But the words are indecipherable.

I return to the hospital at 11 p.m. to find Ayo alone in the TV room. The nurses have told her that Matthew is out of surgery and in recovery.

'The surgeons say it went well,' she says. 'They are pleased with the outcome. They removed more than 90 per cent of the cyst.'

'That's great,' I say. 'What about the remainder?'

'Apparently it was attached too much to the part of the brain they don't want to damage, so they decided to leave it.'

'OK. And no craniotomy?' I ask.

'No, just endoscope.'

This is all very good news, but it doesn't say anything about his condition. I can't let myself assume anything. Until we see him, we won't know.

'They said it shouldn't be too long now,' says Ayo.

An hour passes. 'This is taking too long,' says Ayo. She finds a nurse, who says she will make a call. A few minutes later the nurse waves from where she stands, a little way down the corridor: 'Matthew is on his way.' Another hour passes and we begin to wonder what can be happening. The sky is entirely dark outside and the ward is almost silent. And then there is movement at the end of the corridor: a bed is pushed past and into one of the side wards. We walk down and turn into the room, but a nurse waves us off. 'Give us a few minutes,' he says softly.

We sit again, but this time the delay is short and the nurse calls us back moments later.

I can see Matthew moving from across the ward, and as we approach it's clear that he is awake. Standing next to the bed I am suddenly acutely aware of his body, his physical presence, the weight of him. The cotton rustles as he twists, and as he moves his hands I see they are tangled in the pale lines of the heart monitor, like he is surfacing from deep water, snagged in weeds. His head turns towards us and his breath is sudden, frosting the inside of the transparent oxygen mask that covers his mouth. He clears his throat with a deep, vital sound. He's been intubated. He will be sore. His eyes lock with mine. His voice is thick, trapped by the mask, but his words are full of urgency: 'How did it go?'

And right away I know the answer.

Acknowledgements

I owe special thanks to my friend Andy Sewell for his patient support over many years, and for saying 'do that' when the idea for this book first came up. For early encouragement and feedback I'm also indebted to Juliet Brooke and Kate Murray-Browne. For even earlier encouragement I want to thank Wes White. I'm grateful for the efforts of Will Francis, without whom this book wouldn't have existed, and for those of Juliet Annan, without whom it would have been a far lesser thing. I owe Christina Petrie a great professional debt for the rigour and inspiration she brought to Headway East London's life stories project, *Who are You Now?*, from which I drew freely in writing this book. What I owe her personally is hard to describe and perhaps impossible to repay – but I'll keep trying.

For reading and thinking, my thanks to Natalie Smith, Caroline Pretty, Laura Owens, Ellie Smith, Assallah Tahir and Bryn Davies. For irreplaceable technical and moral assistance: Nora Brennan, Juliet Britton, Will Barker, Ricky Yau and Ernest Aduwa. For being a real friend, Matthew Jones Chesters.

I need to thank Matthew, Danny and Liah, and the other survivors described in this book. Their names, along with some other details, have been changed for the sake of privacy but otherwise they have encouraged me to be bold in telling their stories. For their openness I must also thank the families of those I've written about, as well as Matthew's many wonderful friends for helping me piece together his life before injury. At Headway East London I'm obliged to Tony Bonfil and Miriam Lantsbury, not to mention the rest of the team, for supporting this project and for staying with the trouble.

This book is dedicated to everyone at Headway East London and to the memory of Meg Platts-Mills (also known as Maggie Makepeace).